HESI

ADMISSION ASSESSMENT

Exam Review

EDITION **3**

Editors

Sandra Upchurch, PhD, RN, Director of Curriculum, Review and Testing/HESI

Billie Sharp, Content Manager, Elsevier Health Sciences

Contributing Authors

Mark Basi, MA

Billy R. Glass, AS, BS, DVM

Janice Grams, MA

James Johnston, PhD, RT(R) (CV)

Daniel J. Matusiak, EdD

Amy Rickles, MA

Reviewers

Joan Becker, MA, BSN, RN

Laura C. Bevis, MSN, APRN, FNP, ACNP

Diane Davis, PhD, MLS, SC, SLS (ASCP)^{CM}

Michael Harman

Rebecca Hickey, RN

Kathleen Geiger Hoover, MSN(R), PhD, RN

Janice Grams, MA

Mark Matusiak, BS

Deborah R. Murphy, MSN, RN

Stacey Gerard Thater, MS

Susan A. Weitzel, MN, RN

Gary Kenneth Windler, Jr., BSc, PhD

The editors and publisher would like to acknowledge the following individuals for their contributions to previous editions.

Editors

Donna Boyd

Elizabeth Saccoman, BA

Contributing Authors

Louise Ables, MS

Phil Dickison, PhD, RN

Jean Flick, MS, RN

Mary Hinds, PhD, RN

Judy Hyland, MS, RN

Susan Morrison, PhD, RN

Bernice Rohlich, MS

John Tollett, BS

Deborah L. Walker, MS

Sherry Lutz Zivley, PhD

ELSEVIER

3251 Riverport Lane
St. Louis, Missouri 63043

ADMISSION ASSESSMENT EXAM REVIEW   ISBN: 978-1-4557-0333-3

International Standard Book Number: 978-1-4557-0333-3

Content Manager: Billie Sharp
Freelance Developmental Editor: Betsy McCormac
Publishing Services Manager: Catherine Jackson
Senior Project Manager: David Stein
Design Direction: Margaret Reid

Printed in Canada

Last digit is the print number: 9   8   7   6   5   4   3

PREFACE

Congratulations on purchasing the *HESI Admission Assessment Exam Review*. This study guide was developed based on the HESI Admission Assessment Exam and is designed to assist students in preparation for entrance into higher education in a variety of health-related professions. Test items on the HESI Admission Assessment Exam are not specifically derived from this study guide; however, the content contained in the study guide provides an overview of the subjects tested on the Admission Assessment Exam and is meant to guide students' preparation for the exam. The *HESI Admission Assessment Exam Review* is written at the high school and beginning college levels and offers the basic knowledge that is necessary to be successful on the Admission Assessment Exam.

The HESI Admission Assessment consists of 10 different exams—eight academically oriented exams and two personally oriented exams. The academically oriented subjects consist of

- Mathematics
- Reading Comprehension
- Vocabulary
- Grammar
- Biology
- Chemistry
- Anatomy and Physiology
- Physics

The chapters include conversion tables and practice problems in the Mathematics chapter; step-by-step explanations in the Reading Comprehension and Grammar chapters; a substantial list of words used in health professions in the Vocabulary chapter; rationales and sample questions in the Biology, Chemistry, and Physics chapters; and helpful terminology in the Anatomy and Physiology chapter. Also included throughout the exam review are "HESI Hint" boxes, which are designed to offer students a suggestion, an example, or a reminder pertaining to a specific topic.

The personally oriented exams consist of a Learning Style assessment and a Personality Profile. These exams are intended to offer students insights about their study habits, learning preferences, and dispositions relating to academic achievement. Students generally like to take these exams for the purpose of personal insight and discussion. Because each of the exams takes only approximately 15 minutes to complete, the school may include them in their administration of the Admission Assessment Exam.

Schools can choose to administer any one or all of these exams provided by the Admission Assessment. For example, programs that do not require biology, chemistry, anatomy and physiology, or physics for entry into the program would not administer those Admission Assessment science-oriented exams.

The HESI Admission Assessment Exam has been used by colleges, universities, and health-related institutions as part of the selection and placement process for applicants and newly admitted students for approximately 10 years.

Study Hints

It is always a good idea to prepare for any exam. When you begin to study for the Admission Assessment Exam, make sure you allocate adequate time and do not feel rushed. Set up a schedule that provides an hour or two each day to review material in the *HESI Admission Assessment Exam Review*. Mark the time you set aside on a calendar to remind yourself when to study each day. Review the material for each section in the Admission Assessment Exam Review that is relevant to your particular field of the healthcare professions. Complete the review questions at the end of each chapter. Then complete the corresponding Practice Test in the Appendix. If you are having trouble with the review questions or the Practice Test for a particular section, review that content in the study guide again. It may also be helpful to go back to your textbook and class notes for additional review.

Test-Taking Hints

1. Read each question carefully and completely. Make sure you understand what the question is asking.
2. Identify the key words or phrases in the question. These words or phrases will provide critical information about how to answer the question.
3. Rephrase the question in your words.
   a. Ask yourself, "What is the question really asking?"
   b. Eliminate nonessential information from the question.
   c. Sometimes writers use terminology that may be unfamiliar to you. Do not be confused by a new writing style.
4. Rule out options (if they are presented).
   a. Read all of the responses completely.
   b. Rule out any options that are clearly incorrect.
   c. Mentally mark through incorrect options in your head.
   d. Differentiate between the remaining options, considering your knowledge of the subject.
5. Computer tests do not allow an option for skipping questions and returning to them later. Practice answering every question as it appears.

Do not second-guess yourself. TRUST YOUR ANSWERS.

CONTENTS

1 MATHEMATICS, 1

Basic Addition and Subtraction, 2
Basic Multiplication (Whole Numbers), 4
Basic Division (Whole Numbers), 6
Decimals, 8
Fractions, 13
Multiplication of Fractions, 19
Division of Fractions, 21
Changing Fractions to Decimals, 23
Changing Decimals to Fractions, 25
Ratios and Proportions, 26
Percentages, 28
Regular Time versus Military Time, 32
Algebra, 33
Helpful Information to Memorize, 35
Answers to Sample Problems, 36

2 READING COMPREHENSION, 42

Identifying the Main Idea, 43
Identifying Supporting Details, 43
Finding the Meaning of Words in Context, 43
Identifying a Writer's Purpose and Tone, 44
Distinguishing between Fact and Opinion, 45
Making Logical Inferences, 45
Summarizing, 45

3 VOCABULARY, 48

4 GRAMMAR, 55

Eight Parts of Speech, 56
Nine Important Terms to Understand, 58
Ten Common Grammatical Mistakes, 59
Four Suggestions for Success, 62
Fifteen Troublesome Word Pairs, 62
Summary, 65

5 BIOLOGY, 67

Biology Basics, 68
Water, 68
Biologic Molecules, 68
Metabolism, 69
The Cell, 69
Cellular Respiration, 72
Photosynthesis, 73
Cellular Reproduction, 73
Genetics, 75
DNA, 77

6 CHEMISTRY, 81

Scientific Notation, the Metric System, and
Temperature Scales, 82
Atomic Structure and the Periodic Table, 83
Chemical Equations, 85
Reaction Rates, Equilibrium, and
Reversibility, 86
Solutions and Solution Concentrations, 86
Chemical Reactions, 87
Stoichiometry, 88
Oxidation and Reduction, 89
Acids and Bases, 90
Nuclear Chemistry, 90
Biochemistry, 91

7 ANATOMY AND PHYSIOLOGY, 96

General Terminology, 97
Histology, 97
Mitosis and Meiosis, 98
Skin, 98
Skeletal System, 98
Muscular System, 100
Nervous System, 101
Endocrine System, 102
Circulatory System, 104
Respiratory System, 104
Digestive System, 105
Urinary System, 107
Reproductive System, 108

8 PHYSICS, 112

Nature of Motion, 113
Acceleration, 113
Projectile Motion, 114
Newton's Laws of Motion, 115
Friction, 116
Rotation, 116
Uniform Circular Motion, 117

Kinetic Energy and Potential Energy, 118
Linear Momentum and Impulse, 118
Universal Gravitation, 119
Waves and Sound, 119
Light, 121
Optics, 123
Atomic Structure, 123
The Nature of Electricity, 124
Magnetism and Electricity, 126

APPENDIXES, 127

A. Mathematics Practice Test, 127
B. Reading Comprehension Practice Test, 131
C. Vocabulary Practice Test, 137
D. Grammar Practice Test, 143
E. Biology Practice Test, 148
F. Chemistry Practice Test, 152
G. Anatomy and Physiology Practice Test, 156
H. Physics Practice Test, 160

GLOSSARY, 164

MATHEMATICS

1

M embers of the health professions use math every day to calculate medication dosages, radiation limits, nutritional needs, mental status, intravenous drip rates, intake and output, and a host of other requirements related to their clients. Safe and effective care is the goal of all who work in the health professions. Therefore it is essential that students entering the health professions be able to understand and make calculations using whole numbers, fractions, decimals, and percentages.

The purpose of this chapter is to review the addition, subtraction, multiplication, and division of whole numbers, fractions, decimals, and percentages. Basic algebra skills will also be reviewed: evaluating expressions, and solving for a specific variable. Mastery of these basic mathematic functions is an integral step toward a career in the health professions.

CHAPTER OUTLINE

Basic Addition and
    Subtraction
Basic Multiplication (Whole
    Numbers)
Basic Division (Whole
    Numbers)
Decimals
Fractions

Multiplication of Fractions
Division of Fractions
Changing Fractions to
    Decimals
Changing Decimals to
    Fractions
Ratios and Proportions
Percentages

Regular Time versus Military
    Time
Algebra
Helpful Information to
    Memorize
Answers to Sample
    Problems

KEY TERMS

Common Denominator
Constant
Denominator
Digit
Dividend
Divisor
Exponent
Expression
Factor

Fraction Bar
Improper Fraction
Least Common Denominator
Numerator
Percent
Place Value
Product
Proper Fraction
Proportion

Quotient
Ratio
Reciprocals
Remainder
Terminating
    Decimal
Variable

Basic Addition and Subtraction

Vocabulary

Digit: Any number 1 through 9 and 0 (e.g., the number 7 is a digit).
Place Value: The value of the position of a digit in a number (e.g., in the number 321, the number 2 is in the "tens" position).

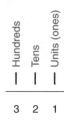

(From Ogden SJ, Fluharty LK: *Calculation of drug dosages: A work text,* ed 9, St. Louis, 2012, Elsevier/Mosby.)

Basic Addition

Example 1

462 + 133

$$\begin{array}{r} 462 \\ + 133 \\ \hline 595 \end{array}$$

Steps

1. Line up the **digits** according to **place value.**
2. Add the digits starting from right to left:
   - Ones: $2 + 3 = 5$
   - Tens: $6 + 3 = 9$
   - Hundreds: $4 + 1 = 5$

Addition with Regrouping

Example 2

835 + 559

$$\begin{array}{r} \overset{1}{8}35 \\ + 559 \\ \hline 1{,}394 \end{array}$$

Steps

1. Line up the digits according to place value.
2. Add:
   - Ones: $5 + 9 = 14$
     - Carry the 1 to the tens place, which is one place to the left.

- Tens: $1 + 3 + 5 = 9$
- Hundreds: $8 + 5 = 13$

Basic Subtraction

Subtraction provides the difference between two numbers.

HESI Hint

It may be easier to solve a subtraction problem by first rewriting it vertically.

Example 1

$5,234 - 4,112$

$$\begin{array}{r} 5,234 \\ -\ 4,112 \\ \hline 1,122 \end{array}$$

Steps

1. Line up the digits according to place value.
2. Subtract:
   - Ones: $4 - 2 = 2$
   - Tens: $3 - 1 = 2$
   - Hundreds: $2 - 1 = 1$
   - Thousands: $5 - 4 = 1$

Subtraction with Regrouping

HESI Hint

Remember, if the number to subtract is not a positive number, you must borrow, or regroup, from one place value to a lower place value.

Example 2

$457 - 29$

$$\begin{array}{r} {}^{4}\ {}^{17} \\ 4\,\cancel{5}\,\cancel{7} \\ -2\ 9 \\ \hline 4\ 2\ 8 \end{array}$$

Steps

1. Align the digits according to place value.
2. Subtract:
   - Ones: $7 - 9$
     - Must borrow 1 from the 5 in the tens place: $17 - 9 = 8$
   - Tens: $4 - 2 = 2$
   - Hundreds: $4 - 0 = 4$

SAMPLE PROBLEMS

Add or subtract each of the following problems as indicated.

1. $1,803 + 156 =$
2. $835 + 145 =$
3. $1,372 + 139 =$

4. $123 + 54 + 23 =$
5. $673 - 241 =$
6. $547 - 88 =$
7. $222 - 114 =$
8. $12,478 - 467 =$
9. Jeff walks 5 miles west then turns north and walks 8 miles. How far has Jeff walked?
10. Julie picks 26 tomatoes from the tomato plants in her garden. She gives seven tomatoes to her next-door neighbor. How many tomatoes does Julie have now?

Basic Multiplication (Whole Numbers)

The process of multiplication is essentially repeated addition.

Vocabulary

Product: The answer to a multiplication problem.

HESI Hint

Remember, the placeholders help keep the problem aligned. If you do not skip a space, the answer will be incorrect. Below is an example of a well-aligned problem.

$$
\begin{array}{r}
24571 \\
\times\ 1233 \\
\hline
73713 \rightarrow \text{Ones} \\
737130 \rightarrow \text{Tens} \\
4914200 \rightarrow \text{Hundreds} \\
+24571000 \rightarrow \text{Thousands} \\
\hline
30,296,043
\end{array}
$$

Example 1

23×5

$$
\begin{array}{r}
\overset{1}{2}3 \\
\times\ 5 \\
\hline
115
\end{array}
$$

Steps

1. Multiply one digit at a time.
2. Multiply 5×23.
   - Ones: $5 \times 3 = 15$
     Carry the 1 to the tens place, and write the 5 in the ones place.
   - Tens: $5 \times 2 = 10 + 1 = 11$

Example 2

623×45

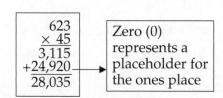

$$
\begin{array}{r}
623 \\
\times\ 45 \\
\hline
3,115 \\
+24,920 \\
\hline
28,035
\end{array}
$$

Zero (0) represents a placeholder for the ones place

Steps

1. Multiply 623×5.
   - $5 \times 3 = 15$
   - $5 \times 2 = 10 + 1$ (carried over) $= 11$
   - $5 \times 6 = 30 + 1$ (carried over) $= 31$ (does not need to be carried)
2. Multiply 623×4 (remember to line up the ones digit with the 4 by using zero as a placeholder).
   - $4 \times 3 = 12$
   - $4 \times 2 = 8 + 1 = 9$
   - $4 \times 6 = 24$
3. Add the two products together.
   - $3{,}115 + 24{,}920 = 28{,}035$ (the final **product**)

Example 3

301×451

$$
\begin{array}{r}
301 \\
\times\ 451 \\
\hline
301 \\
15{,}050 \\
+\ 120{,}400 \\
\hline
135{,}751
\end{array}
$$

Steps

1. Multiply 301×1.
   - $1 \times 1 = 1$
   - $1 \times 0 = 0$
   - $1 \times 3 = 3$
2. Multiply 301×5.
   - $5 \times 1 = 5$ (remember to use a zero for a placeholder)
   - $5 \times 0 = 0$
   - $5 \times 3 = 15$
3. Multiply 301×4.
   - $4 \times 1 = 4$
   - $4 \times 0 = 0$
   - $4 \times 3 = 12$
4. Add the three products together.
   - $301 + 15{,}050 + 120{,}400 = 135{,}751$ (the final **product**)

SAMPLE PROBLEMS

Multiply each of the following problems as indicated.

1. $846 \times 7 =$
2. $325 \times 6 =$
3. $653 \times 12 =$
4. $806 \times 55 =$
5. $795 \times 14 =$
6. $999 \times 22 =$
7. $582 \times 325 =$
8. $9438 \times 165 =$
9. Jan is preparing an examination for 29 students. Each student will have 30 questions, with no student having duplicate questions. How many questions will Jan need to prepare?
10. John is ordering lunch for the volunteers at the hospital. There are 12 units in the hospital, with 15 volunteers in each unit. How many lunches will John need to order?

Basic Division (Whole Numbers)

Vocabulary

Dividend: The number being divided.
Divisor: The number by which the dividend is divided.
Quotient: The answer to a division problem.
Remainder: The portion of the dividend that is not evenly divisible by the divisor.

HESI Hint

$$\begin{array}{r} 9 \\ 5\overline{)45} \end{array}$$

The 45 represents the **dividend** (the number being divided), the 5 represents the **divisor** (the number by which the dividend is divided), and the 9 represents the **quotient** (the answer to the division problem). It is best not to leave a division problem with a **remainder,** but to end it as a fraction or decimal instead. To make the problem into a decimal, add a decimal point and zeros at the end of the dividend and continue. If a remainder continues to occur, round to the hundredths place.

Example:

233.547 → 233.55 (the 7 rounds the 4 to a 5)

Example 1

40 ÷ 8

Steps

1. Set up the problem.
2. Use a series of multiplication and subtraction problems to solve a division problem.
3. 8 × ? = 40
   - Multiply: 8 × 5 = 40
   - Subtract: 40 − 40 = 0
   - The quotient (or answer) is 5.

Example 2

672 ÷ 6

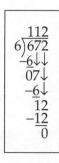

Steps
1. Set up the problem.
2. Begin with the hundreds place.
   - $6 \times ? = 6$. We know $6 \times 1 = 6$; therefore place the 1 (quotient) above the 6 in the hundreds place (dividend). Place the other 6 under the hundreds place and subtract: $6 - 6 = 0$.
   - Bring down the next number, which is 7; $6 \times ? = 7$. There is no number that can be multiplied by 6 that will equal 7 exactly, so try to get as close as possible without going over 7. Use $6 \times 1 = 6$ and set it up just like the last subtraction problem: $7 - 6 = 1$.
   - Bring down the 2 from the dividend, which results in the number 12 (the 1 came from the remainder of $7 - 6 = 1$).
   - $6 \times ? = 12; ? = 2$. The two becomes the next number in the quotient. $12 - 12 = 0$. There is not a remainder.
   - The quotient (or answer) is 112.

Example 3

$174 \div 5$

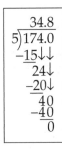

Steps
1. Set up the problem.
2. 5 does not divide into 1 but does divide into 17.
3. $5 \times 3 = 15$. Write the 3 in the quotient. (It is written above the 7 in 17 because that is the last digit in the number.)
   - $5 \times 3 = 15$
   - $17 - 15 = 2$
4. Bring the 4 down. Combine the 2 (remainder from $17 - 15$) and 4 to create 24.
5. Five does not divide evenly into 24; therefore try to get close without going over.
   - $5 \times 4 = 20$
   - $24 - 20 = 4$
6. There is a remainder of 4, but there is not a number left in the dividend. Add a decimal point and zeros and continue to divide.
7. The quotient (or answer) is 34.8 (thirty-four and eight tenths).

SAMPLE PROBLEMS

Divide in each of the following problems as indicated.
1. $132 \div 11 =$
2. $9,618 \div 3 =$
3. $2,466 \div 2 =$
4. $325 \div 13 =$
5. $5,024 \div 8 =$

6. $3,705 \div 5 =$
7. $859 \div 4 =$
8. $6,987 \div 7 =$
9. There are 225 pieces of candy in a large jar. Ben wants to give the 25 campers in his group an even amount of candy. How many pieces of candy will each camper receive?
10. Edie has 132 tulip bulbs. She wants to plant all of the tulip bulbs in 12 rows. How many tulip bulbs will Edie plant in each row?

Decimals

A decimal pertains to tenths or to the number 10.

Vocabulary

Place value: Regarding decimals, numbers to the right of the decimal point have different terms from the whole numbers to the left of the decimal point. Each digit in a number occupies a position called a **place value**.

HESI Hint

Remember, whole numbers are written to the left of the decimal point and place values are written to the right of the decimal point. Line the numbers up vertically before solving the problem.

Addition and Subtraction of Decimals

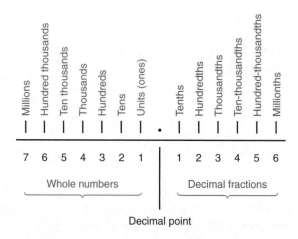

(From Ogden SJ, Fluharty LK: *Calculation of drug dosages: A work text*, ed 9, St. Louis, 2012, Elsevier/Mosby.)

HESI Hint

The word "and" stands for the decimal when writing a number in words.
Example: 5.7 (five *and* seven tenths)

Example 1

$2.6 + 3.1$

$$\begin{array}{r} 2.6 \\ + 3.1 \\ \hline 5.7 \end{array}$$

Steps

1. Align the decimal points.
2. Add the tenths together: $6 + 1 = 7$
3. Add the ones together: $3 + 2 = 5$
4. Final answer: 5.7 (five and seven tenths).

Example 2

$5 + 12.34$

$$\begin{array}{r} 12.34 \\ + 5.00 \\ \hline 17.34 \end{array}$$

Steps

1. Align the decimal points.
   - It might be difficult to align the 5 because it does not have a decimal point. Remember that after the ones place, there is a decimal point. To help with organization, add zeros (placeholders). Example: $5 = 5.00$
2. Add the hundredths: $4 + 0 = 4$
3. Add the tenths: $3 + 0 = 3$
4. Add the ones: $2 + 5 = 7$
5. Add the tens: $1 + 0 = 1$
6. Final answer: 17.34 (seventeen and thirty-four hundredths).

Example 3

$7.21 - 4.01$

$$\begin{array}{r} 7.21 \\ - 4.01 \\ \hline 3.20 \end{array}$$

Steps

1. Align the decimal points.
2. Subtract the hundredths: $1 - 1 = 0$
3. Subtract the tenths: $2 - 0 = 2$
4. Subtract the ones: $7 - 4 = 3$
5. Final answer: 3.20 (three and twenty hundredths).

Example 4

$12 - 8.99$

$$\begin{array}{r} {}^{1}{}^{9}{}^{10} \\ 1\cancel{2}.\cancel{0}\cancel{0} \\ -8.9\cancel{9} \\ \hline 3.01 \end{array}$$

Steps

1. Align the decimal points.
2. Because 12 is a whole number, add a decimal point and zeros.
3. $0.00 - 0.99$ cannot be subtracted; therefore 1 must be borrowed from the 12 and regrouped.
4. The ones become 1, the tenths become 9, and the hundredths become 10.
5. Subtract the hundredths: $10 - 9 = 1$
6. Subtract the tenths: $9 - 9 = 0$
7. Subtract the ones: $11 - 8 = 3$
   - 1 was borrowed from the tens in order to subtract the 8.
8. Final answer: 3.01 (three and one hundredth).

Solve each of the following decimal problems as indicated.
1. $9.2 + 7.55 =$
2. $2.258 + 64.58 =$
3. $892.2 + 56 =$
4. $22 + 3.26 =$
5. $8.5 + 7.55 + 14 =$
6. $18 - 7.55 =$
7. $31.84 - 2.430 =$
8. $21.36 - 8.79 =$
9. Bill has 2.5 vacation days left for the rest of the year and 1.25 sick days left. If Bill uses all of his sick days and his vacation days, how many days will he have off work?
10. Erin has 6.25 peach pies. She gives Rose 3.75 of the peach pies. How many pies does Erin have left?

Multiplication of Decimals

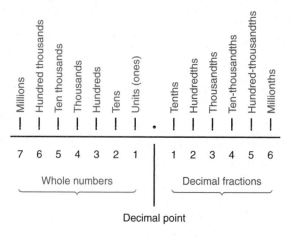

(From Ogden SJ, Fluharty LK: *Calculation of drug dosages: A work text*, ed 9, St. Louis, 2012, Elsevier/Mosby.)

Example 1

75.7×2.1

$$
\begin{array}{r}
75.7 \\
\times\ 2.1 \\
\hline
757 \\
+\ 15140 \\
\hline
158.97
\end{array}
$$

1 decimal place
+ 1 decimal place
_____
2 decimal places

Move the decimal point two places to the left in the final product.

Steps

1. Multiply 757×21 (do not worry about the decimal point until the final product has been calculated).
2. Starting from the right, count the decimal places in both numbers and add together (two decimal places).
3. Move to the left two places, and then place the decimal point.

Example 2

0.002×3.4

$$
\begin{array}{r}
0.002 \\
\times \quad 3.4 \\
\hline
0008 \\
+ \ 00060 \\
\hline
0.0068
\end{array}
$$

| 3 decimal places |
| + 1 decimal place |
| 4 decimal places |
| Move four places to the left. |

Steps

1. Multiply 2 × 34.
2. Starting from the right, count the decimal places in both numbers and add together (four decimal places).
3. Move to the left four places, and then place the decimal.

Example 3

3.41×7

$$
\begin{array}{r}
3.41 \\
\times \quad 7 \\
\hline
23.87
\end{array}
$$

| 2 decimal places |
| + 0 decimal places |
| 2 decimal places |
| Move two places to the left. |

Steps

1. Multiply 341 × 7.
2. Starting from the right, count the decimal places in both numbers and add together (two decimal places).
3. Move to the left two places, and then place the decimal point.

SAMPLE PROBLEMS

Multiply the decimals in the following problems as indicated.

1. $0.003 \times 4.23 =$
2. $98.26 \times 8 =$
3. $8.03 \times 2.1 =$
4. $250.1 \times 25 =$
5. $0.1364 \times 2.11 =$
6. $8.23 \times 4 =$
7. $0.058 \times 64.2 =$
8. $794.23 \times .001 =$
9. Jenny lost 3.2 lb each month for 6 months. How much weight has Jenny lost?
10. Richard wants to make 2.5 batches of sugar cookies. One batch calls for 1.75 cups of sugar. How many cups of sugar will Richard need for 2.5 batches of cookies?

Division of Decimals

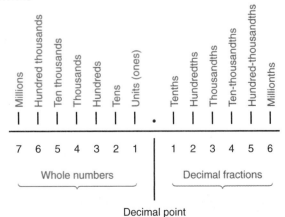

(From Ogden SJ, Fluharty LK: *Calculation of drug dosages: A work text*, ed 9, St. Louis, 2012, Elsevier/Mosby.)

Example 1

$34 \div 2.5$

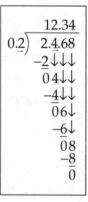

$$
\begin{array}{r}
13.6 \\
2.\underline{5}\,)\,\overline{34.\underline{0}.0} \\
-25\downarrow\downarrow \\
\hline
90\downarrow \\
-75\downarrow \\
\hline
150 \\
-150 \\
\hline
0
\end{array}
$$

Steps

1. Set up the division problem.
2. Move the decimal point in 2.5 one place to the right, making it a whole number.
3. What is done to one side must be done to the other side. Move the decimal point one place to the right in 34, making it 340, and then bring the decimal point up into the quotient.
4. Divide normally.
   - $25 \times 1 = 25$
   - Subtract: $34 - 25 = 9$
   - Bring down the zero to make 90.
   - $25 \times 3 = 75$. This is as close to 90 as possible without going over.
   - Subtract: $90 - 75 = 15$
   - Add a zero to the dividend and bring it down to the 15, making it 150.
   - $25 \times 6 = 150$
   - $150 - 150 = 0$
5. The quotient is 13.6.

Example 2

$2.468 \div 0.2$

$$
\begin{array}{r}
12.34 \\
0.\underline{2}\,)\,\overline{2.\underline{4}.68} \\
-2\downarrow\downarrow\downarrow \\
\hline
04\downarrow\downarrow \\
-4\downarrow\downarrow \\
\hline
06\downarrow \\
-6\downarrow \\
\hline
08 \\
-8 \\
\hline
0
\end{array}
$$

Steps

1. Set up the division problem.
2. Move the decimal point in 0.2 over one place to the right, making it a whole number. 0.2 is now 2.

3. Move the same number of spaces in the dividend. 2.468 is now 24.68.
4. Bring the decimal point up to the quotient in the new position.
5. Divide normally.

Example 3

0.894 ÷ 0.05

```
              17.88
      _____
0.05) 0.89.40
      −5↓↓↓
       39↓↓
      −35↓↓
        44↓
       −40↓
         40
        −40
          0
```

Steps

1. Set up the division problem.
2. Move the decimal point in the divisor until it is a whole number. 0.05 is now 5.
3. Move the decimal point in the dividend the same number of spaces as was moved in the divisor. 0.894 is now 89.4.
4. Divide normally.

SAMPLE PROBLEMS

Divide the decimals in the following problems as indicated.
1. 48 ÷ 0.4 =
2. 144 ÷ 0.6 =
3. 3.75 ÷ 0.4 =
4. 56.2 ÷ 0.2 =
5. 2.6336 ÷ 0.32 =
6. 591 ÷ 0.3 =
7. 0.72 ÷ 0.8 =
8. 0.132 ÷ 0.11 =
9. Stewart has 56 acres of land. He wants to divide the land into plots of 0.25 acres. How many plots of land will Stewart have after he divides the 56 acres?
10. Donna has 4.2 liters of fertilizer. If each pecan tree needs 0.7 liters of fertilizer and Donna uses all of the fertilizer, how many pecan trees does Donna have?

Fractions

In mathematics, a fraction is a way to express a part in relation to the total.

Vocabulary

Numerator: The top number in a fraction.
Denominator: The bottom number in a fraction.

Fraction Bar: The line between the numerator and denominator. The bar is another symbol for division.

Factor: A number that divides evenly into another number.

Least Common Denominator: The smallest multiple that two numbers share.

Improper Fraction: A fraction where the numerator is larger than the denominator.

Proper Fraction: A fraction where the denominator is larger than the numerator.

Common Denominator: Two or more fractions having the same denominator.

Reciprocals: Pairs of numbers that equal 1 when multiplied together.

Terminating Decimal: A decimal that is not continuous.

$$\frac{\text{Numerator (part)}}{\text{Denominator (whole)}} \text{ Fraction bar}$$

HESI Hint

- The **numerator** is the top number of the fraction. It represents the part or pieces.
- The **denominator** is the bottom number of the fraction. It represents the total or whole amount.
- The **fraction bar** is the line that separates the numerator and the denominator.

Reducing Fractions Using the Greatest Common Factor

A **factor** is a number that divides evenly into another number.

Factors of 12:

- $1 \times 12 = 12$
- $2 \times 6 = 12$
- $3 \times 4 = 12$

12 {1, 2, 3, 4, 6, 12}: Listing the factors helps determine the greatest common factor between two or more numbers.

$$\frac{1}{2} = \frac{2}{4}, \frac{3}{6}, \frac{4}{8}, \frac{5}{10}, \frac{6}{12}, \frac{7}{14}, \frac{8}{16}, \frac{9}{18}, \frac{10}{20}$$

All represent one-half.

Reducing fractions can also be called reducing a fraction to its lowest terms or simplest form.

$$1 = \frac{1}{1}, \frac{2}{2}, \frac{3}{3}, \frac{4}{4}, \frac{5}{5}, \frac{6}{6}, \frac{7}{7}, \frac{8}{8}, \frac{9}{9}, \frac{10}{10}$$

Example 1

Reduce $\frac{7}{21}$

Factors of 7 and 21:

7 {1, **7**}

21 {1, 3, **7**, 21}

The greatest common factor is 7; therefore divide the numerator and denominator by 7.

$$\frac{7}{21} \div \frac{7}{7} = \frac{1}{3}$$

Example 2

Reduce $\frac{12}{20}$

Factors of 12 and 20:

12 {1, 2, 3, **4**, 6, 12}
20 {1, 2, **4**, 5, 10, 20}

The greatest common factor is 4 (they do have 1 and 2 in common, but the greatest factor is best).

$$\frac{12}{20} \div \frac{4}{4} = \frac{3}{5}$$

Least Common Denominator

The **least common denominator** (LCD) is the smallest multiple that two numbers share. Determining the LCD is an essential step in the addition, subtraction, and ordering of fractions.

Example 1

Find the LCD for $\frac{3}{4}$ and $\frac{7}{9}$.

Steps

1. List the multiples (multiplication tables) of each denominator.
   - $4: 4 \times 1 = 4, 4 \times 2 = 8, 4 \times 3 = 12, 4 \times 4 = 16, 4 \times 5 = 20, 4 \times 6 = 24, 4 \times 7 = 28, 4 \times 8 = 32, 4 \times 9 = 36, 4 \times 10 = 40$
   - 4 {4, 8, 12, 16, 20, 24, 28, 32, 36, 40}—this will be the standard form throughout for listing multiples.
   - 9 {9, 18, 27, 36, 45, 54, 63, 72, 81, 90}
2. Compare each for the least common multiple.
   - 4 {4, 8, 12, 16, 20, 24, 28, 32, **36**, 40}
   - 9 {9, 18, 27, **36**, 45, 54, 63, 72, 81, 90}
3. The LCD between 4 and 9 is 36 ($4 \times 9 = 36$ and $9 \times 4 = 36$).

Example 2

Find the LCD for $\frac{3}{12}$ and $\frac{1}{8}$.

Steps

1. List the multiples of each denominator, and find the common multiples.
   - 12 {12, **24**, 36, 48, 60, 72, 84, 96, 108, 120}
   - 8 {8, 16, **24**, 32, 40, 48, 56, 64, 72, 80}
2. The LCD between 12 and 8 is 24 ($12 \times 2 = 24$ and $8 \times 3 = 24$).

Changing Improper Fractions into Mixed Numbers

An **improper fraction** occurs when the numerator is larger than the denominator. An improper fraction should be reduced and made into a mixed number.

Example

$$\frac{17}{5} \rightarrow 5\overline{)17} \begin{array}{c} 3 \\ 15 \\ \hline 2 \end{array} \rightarrow 3\frac{2}{5}$$

Steps

1. Turn an improper fraction into a mixed number through division. (The top number [numerator] goes in the box [17]; the bottom number [denominator] stays out [5].)
2. The 3 becomes the whole number.

3. The remainder (2) becomes the numerator.
4. The denominator stays the same.

Changing Mixed Numbers into Improper Fractions

A mixed number has a whole number and fraction combined.
Example

$$5\frac{2}{3} \rightarrow 5\frac{+2}{\times 3} = (5 \times 3) + 2 = 17 \rightarrow \frac{17}{3}$$

Steps

1. To make a mixed number into an improper fraction, multiply the denominator (3) and whole number (5) together, then add the numerator (2).
2. Place this new numerator (17) over the denominator (3), which stays the same in the mixed number.

Addition of Fractions

Addition with Common Denominators
Example

$$\frac{3}{7} + \frac{2}{7} = \frac{5}{7}$$

Steps

1. Add the numerators together: $3 + 2 = 5$.
2. The denominator (7) stays the same. This makes it a **common denominator.**
3. Answer: $\frac{5}{7}$ (five sevenths).

Addition with Unlike Denominators
Example

$$\frac{1}{5} + \frac{7}{10}$$

$$\frac{1 \times 2}{5 \times 2} = \frac{2}{10}$$

$$\frac{7 \times 1}{10 \times 1} = \frac{7}{10}$$

$$\frac{2}{10} + \frac{7}{10} = \frac{9}{10}$$

Steps

1. Find the LCD by listing the multiple of each denominator.
   - 5 (5, **10**, 15, 20, 25, 30)
   - 10 (**10**, 20, 30, 40, 50)
   - The LCD is 10.
2. If the denominator is changed, the numerator must also be changed by the same number. Do this by multiplying the numerator and denominator by the same number.

$$\frac{1 \times 2}{5 \times 2} = \frac{2}{10}$$

3. Because the denominator of the second fraction is 10, no change is necessary.
4. Add the numerators together, and keep the common denominator.
5. Reduce the fraction if necessary.

Addition of Mixed Numbers

Example

$$1\frac{1}{4} + 2\frac{8}{10}$$

$$1\frac{1 \times 5}{4 \times 5} = 1\frac{5}{20}$$

$$2\frac{8 \times 2}{10 \times 2} = 2\frac{16}{20}$$

$$1\frac{5}{20} + 2\frac{16}{20} = 3\frac{21}{20} = 4\frac{1}{20}$$

Steps

1. Find the least common denominator of 4 and 10 by listing the multiples of each.
   - 4 (4, 8, 12, 16, **20**)
   - 10 (10, **20**, 30)
2. Calculate the new numerator of each fraction to correspond to the changed denominator.
3. Add the whole numbers together, and then add the numerators together. Keep the common denominator 20.
4. The numerator is larger than the denominator (improper); change the answer to a mixed number (review vocabulary if necessary).

SAMPLE PROBLEMS

Add the fractions in the following problems as indicated.

1. $\dfrac{1}{12} + \dfrac{5}{12} =$

2. $\dfrac{7}{21} + \dfrac{10}{21} =$

3. $\dfrac{1}{2} + \dfrac{4}{5} =$

4. $\dfrac{5}{7} + \dfrac{3}{14} =$

5. $\dfrac{4}{5} + \dfrac{6}{7} =$

6. $7\dfrac{1}{8} + 2\dfrac{4}{12} =$

7. $5\dfrac{2}{9} + 1\dfrac{2}{9} =$

8. $12\dfrac{1}{21} + 3\dfrac{1}{3} =$

9. Mary is going to make a birthday cake. She will need 1⅔ cups of sugar for the cake and 2½ cups of sugar for the frosting. How many cups of sugar will Mary need for the frosted birthday cake?

10. Greg is installing crown molding on two sides of a room. The length of one wall is 11¾ feet. The length of the other wall is 13⅞ feet. How much crown molding will Greg install in the room?

Subtraction of Fractions

Subtracting Fractions with Common Denominators
Example

$$\frac{7}{9} - \frac{4}{9} = \frac{3}{9} = \frac{1}{3}$$

Steps

1. Subtract the numerators: $(7 - 4 = 3)$
2. Keep the common denominator.
3. Reduce the fraction by dividing by the greatest common factor:

$$\frac{3}{9} \div \frac{3}{3} = \frac{1}{3}$$

Subtracting Fractions with Unlike Denominators

Example

$$\frac{5}{12} - \frac{1}{8} = ?$$

$$\frac{5 \times 2}{12 \times 2} = \frac{10}{24}$$

$$\frac{1 \times 3}{8 \times 3} = \frac{3}{24}$$

$$\frac{10}{24} - \frac{3}{24} = \frac{7}{24}$$

Steps

1. Find the LCD by listing the multiples of each denominator.
   - 12 {12, **24**, 36, 48}
   - 8 {8, 16, **24**, 32}
   - The LCD is 24.
2. Change the numerator to reflect the new denominator. (What is done to the bottom must be done to the top of a fraction.)
3. Subtract the new numerators: $10 - 3 = 7$. The denominator stays the same.

Borrowing from Whole Numbers

Example

$$5\frac{2}{3} - 3\frac{4}{5}$$

$$5\frac{2 \times 5}{3 \times 5} = 5\frac{10}{15}$$

$$^4\cancel{5}\frac{10}{15} + \frac{15}{15} = 4\frac{25}{15}$$

$$3\frac{4 \times 3}{5 \times 3} = 3\frac{12}{15}$$

$$4\frac{25}{15} - 3\frac{12}{15} = 1\frac{13}{15}$$

Steps

1. Find the LCD.
2. Twelve cannot be subtracted from 10; therefore 1 must be borrowed from the whole number, making it 4, and the borrowed 1 must be added to the fraction.
3. Add the original numerator to the borrowed numerator: $10 + 15 = 25$.
4. Now the whole number and the numerator can be subtracted.

HESI Hint

Fractions as a whole:
$$\frac{15}{15} = 1 \text{ (one whole)}$$
Notice in the example under "Borrowing from Whole Numbers" that we added 15 to both the numerator and the denominator. We did this because it is one whole and it is the same denominator.

SAMPLE PROBLEMS

Subtract the fractions in the following problems as indicated.

1. $\dfrac{3}{20} - \dfrac{2}{20} =$

2. $\dfrac{28}{37} - \dfrac{17}{37} =$

3. $\dfrac{17}{25} - \dfrac{3}{5} =$

4. $\dfrac{31}{54} - \dfrac{5}{9} =$

5. $1\dfrac{9}{10} - \dfrac{1}{5} =$

6. $15\dfrac{7}{18} - \dfrac{3}{9} =$

7. $25\dfrac{1}{7} - 12\dfrac{5}{7} =$

8. $30\dfrac{1}{2} - 13\dfrac{3}{4} =$

9. Alan is making a table. The table will be 6½ feet long and 4 feet wide. The board for the table is 7⅞ feet long and 4 feet wide. How much of the board will Alan need to cut off?

10. McKenna has 1⅔ cups of milk. She gives Mark ¾ cup of milk to make a cake. How much milk will McKenna have left?

Multiplication of Fractions

HESI Hint

"Multiplying fractions is no problem. Top times top and bottom times bottom."
To change an improper fraction into a mixed number, divide the numerator by the denominator.

$$\frac{20}{13} \rightarrow 13\overline{)20} \rightarrow 1\frac{7}{13}$$
$$\phantom{\frac{20}{13} \rightarrow 13)}\underline{13}$$
$$\phantom{\frac{20}{13} \rightarrow 13)}07$$

The quotient becomes the whole number. The remainder becomes the numerator, and the denominator stays the same.

Example 1

$$\frac{4}{5} \times \frac{1}{2}$$

$$\frac{4}{5} \times \frac{1}{2} = \frac{4}{10} = \frac{2}{5}$$

Steps

1. Multiply the numerators together: $4 \times 1 = 4$.
2. Multiply the denominators together: $5 \times 2 = 10$.
3. Reduce the product by using the greatest common factor: $\dfrac{4 \div 2}{10 \div 2} = \dfrac{2}{5}$.

Example 2

$$5 \times \frac{4}{13}$$

$$\frac{5}{1} \times \frac{4}{13} = \frac{20}{13} = 1\frac{7}{13}$$

Steps

1. Make the whole number 5 into a fraction by placing a 1 as the denominator.
2. Multiply the numerators: $5 \times 4 = 20$.
3. Multiply the denominators: $1 \times 13 = 13$.
4. Change the improper fraction into a mixed number.

Example 3

$$2\frac{1}{8} \times 7\frac{5}{6}$$

$$2\frac{1}{8} \times 7\frac{5}{6}$$

$$\frac{17}{8} \times \frac{47}{6} = \frac{799}{48}$$

$$\frac{799}{48} = 16\frac{31}{48}$$

Steps

1. Change the mixed numbers into improper fractions.

$$2\frac{+1}{\times 8} = (2 \times 8) + 1 = 17 \rightarrow \frac{17}{8}$$

$$7\frac{+5}{\times 6} = (7 \times 6) + 5 = 47 \rightarrow \frac{47}{6}$$

2. Multiply the numerators and denominators together.
   - $17 \times 47 = 799$ (numerator)
   - $8 \times 6 = 48$ (denominator)
   - Change the improper fraction into a mixed number.

$$\begin{array}{r} 16 \\ 48\overline{)799} \\ \underline{48} \\ 319 \\ \underline{288} \\ 31 \end{array} = 16\frac{31}{48}$$

SAMPLE PROBLEMS

Multiply the following fractions and reduce the product to the lowest common denominator.

1. $\dfrac{3}{5} \times \dfrac{2}{3} =$

2. $\dfrac{7}{9} \times \dfrac{1}{9} =$

3. $6 \times \dfrac{4}{5} =$

4. $1\dfrac{2}{5} \times 5 =$

5. $2\dfrac{1}{7} \times 1\dfrac{3}{4} =$

6. $4\dfrac{4}{5} \times 1\dfrac{4}{6} =$

7. $3\dfrac{1}{3} \times 2 =$

8. $1\dfrac{8}{12} \times 4\dfrac{1}{2} =$

9. Alec has six friends who each give him 2¾ pieces of gum. How many pieces of gum does Alec have now?

10. Rick rides 11⅛ miles in an hour with his bike in second gear going uphill. If Rick rides downhill in fourth gear he goes 2½ times faster. How many miles will Rick go in an hour downhill in fourth gear?

Division of Fractions

HESI Hint

"Dividing fractions, don't ask why, inverse the second fraction and multiply."

Example:

$\dfrac{1}{2} \div \dfrac{3}{8}$ Inverse $\dfrac{3}{8} \rightarrow \dfrac{8}{3}$

Then multiply $\dfrac{1}{2} \times \dfrac{8}{3}$

$\dfrac{3}{8} \rightarrow \dfrac{8}{3} \quad \dfrac{3}{8} \times \dfrac{8}{3} = \dfrac{24}{24} = 1$

These two numbers ($\dfrac{3}{8}$ and $\dfrac{8}{3}$) are **reciprocals** of each other because when they are multiplied together, they equal 1.

Example 1

$\dfrac{1}{2} \div \dfrac{3}{8}$

$\boxed{\begin{array}{c} \dfrac{1}{2} \div \dfrac{3}{8} \\[2mm] \dfrac{1}{2} \times \dfrac{8}{3} = \dfrac{8}{6} \end{array}}$

Steps

1. Inverse (or take the reciprocal) of the second fraction: $\dfrac{3}{8} \rightarrow \dfrac{8}{3}$.
2. Rewrite the new problem and multiply.
   - $1 \times 8 = 8$ (numerator)
   - $2 \times 3 = 6$ (denominator)

Example 2

$1\dfrac{5}{6} \div \dfrac{3}{4}$

$\boxed{\begin{array}{c} 1\dfrac{5}{6} \div \dfrac{3}{4} \\[2mm] \dfrac{11}{6} \div \dfrac{3}{4} \\[2mm] \dfrac{11}{6} \times \dfrac{4}{3} = \dfrac{44}{18} \\[2mm] 2\dfrac{8}{18} = 2\dfrac{4}{9} \end{array}}$

Steps

1. Change the mixed number into an improper fraction: $1\frac{5}{6} = (1 \times 6) + 5 = \frac{11}{6}$.
2. Rewrite the new problem with the improper fraction.
3. Inverse the second fraction.
4. Multiply the numerators and the denominators together.
   - $11 \times 4 = 44$ (numerators)
   - $6 \times 3 = 18$ (denominators)
5. Change the improper fraction into a mixed number. Reduce the mixed number.

Example 3

$12 \div 2\frac{3}{8}$

$$\frac{12}{1} \div \frac{19}{8}$$

$$\frac{12}{1} \times \frac{8}{19} = \frac{96}{19}$$

$$5\frac{1}{19}$$

Steps

1. Change the whole number into a fraction and the mixed number into an improper fraction.
2. Inverse the second fraction.
3. Multiply the numerators and then denominators together.
   - $12 \times 8 = 96$
   - $1 \times 19 = 19$
4. Change the improper fraction into a mixed number.

SAMPLE PROBLEMS

Divide the fractions in the following problems and reduce to the lowest common denominator.

1. $\frac{4}{5} \div \frac{1}{7} =$

2. $\frac{12}{15} \div \frac{3}{5} =$

3. $\frac{7}{8} \div \frac{1}{6} =$

4. $1 \div \frac{1}{5} =$

5. $8 \div \frac{1}{4} =$

6. $2\frac{1}{4} \div \frac{1}{4} =$

7. $10 \div 3\frac{1}{3} =$

8. $12\frac{1}{3} \div 2 =$

9. Danny has 11¼ cups of chocolate syrup. He is going to make chocolate sundaes for his friends. Each sundae will have ¾ cup of chocolate. How many sundaes can Danny make?

10. Jenny has 8⅓ yards of ribbon. She is making bows for her bridesmaids. Each bow has ⅚ yard of ribbon. How many bridesmaids does Jenny have for her wedding?

Changing Fractions to Decimals

HESI Hint

"Top goes in the box, the bottom goes out."
This is a helpful saying in remembering that the numerator is the dividend and the denominator is the divisor.

If the decimal does not terminate, continue to the thousandths place and then round to the hundredths place.

Example:

$7.8666 \rightarrow 7.87$

If the number in the thousandths place is 5 or greater, round the number in the hundredths place to the next higher number.

However, if the number in the thousandths place is less than 5, do not round up the number in the hundredths place.

Example 1

Change $\dfrac{3}{4}$ to a decimal.

$$\begin{array}{r} 0.75 \\ 4\overline{)3.00} \\ -28\downarrow \\ \hline 20 \\ -20 \\ \hline 0 \end{array}$$

Steps

1. Change the fraction into a division problem.
2. Add a decimal point after the 3 and add two zeros.
   • Remember to raise the decimal into the quotient area.
3. The answer is a **terminating decimal** (a decimal that is not continuous); therefore adding additional zeros is not necessary.

Example 2

Change $\dfrac{5}{8}$ to a decimal.

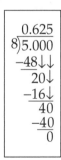

$$\begin{array}{r} 0.625 \\ 8\overline{)5.000} \\ -48\downarrow\downarrow \\ \hline 20\downarrow \\ -16\downarrow \\ \hline 40 \\ -40 \\ \hline 0 \end{array}$$

Steps

1. Change the fraction into a division problem.
2. Add a decimal point after the 5 and add two zeros.
   • Remember to raise the decimal into the quotient area.
3. If there is still a remainder, add another zero to the dividend and bring it down.
4. The decimal terminates at the thousandths place.

Example 3

Change $\frac{2}{3}$ to a decimal.

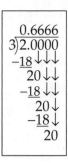

Steps

1. Change the fraction into a division problem.
2. After the 2, add a decimal point and two zeros.
3. The decimal continues (does not terminate); therefore round to the hundredths place: $0.666 \rightarrow 0.67$. (It can also be written as $0.\overline{6}$. The line is placed over the number that repeats.)

Example 4

Change $2\frac{3}{5}$ to a decimal.

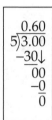

Steps

1. Change the fraction into a division problem.
2. After the 3, add a decimal and two zeros.
3. Place the whole number in front of the decimal: 2.6.

SAMPLE PROBLEMS

Change the following fractions into decimals and round to the nearest thousandth.

1. $\frac{1}{5}$

2. $\frac{2}{5}$

3. $\frac{3}{8}$

4. $\frac{4}{5}$

5. $\frac{1}{3}$

6. $1\frac{1}{2}$

7. $\frac{3}{10}$

8. $2\frac{7}{8}$

9. $11\frac{11}{15}$

10. $\frac{11}{25}$

Changing Decimals to Fractions

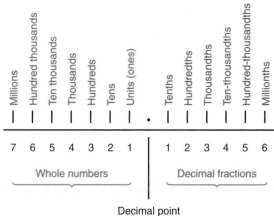

Decimal point

(From Ogden SJ, Fluharty LK: *Calculation of drug dosages: A work text*, ed 9, St. Louis, 2012, Elsevier/Mosby.)

Example 1

Change 0.9 to a fraction.

$$0.9 \rightarrow \frac{9}{10}$$

Steps

Knowing place values makes it very simple to change decimals to fractions.
1. The last digit is located in the tenths place; therefore the 9 becomes the numerator.
2. 10 becomes the denominator.

Example 2

Change 0.02 to a fraction.

$$0.02 \rightarrow \frac{2}{100} = \frac{1}{50}$$

Steps

1. The 2 is located in the hundredths place.
2. The numerator becomes 2, and 100 becomes the denominator.
3. Reduce the fraction.

Example 3

Change 0.25 to a fraction.

$$0.25 \rightarrow \frac{25}{100} = \frac{1}{4}$$

Steps

1. Always look at the last digit in the decimal. In this example the 5 is located in the hundredths place.
2. The numerator becomes 25, and 100 becomes the denominator.
3. Reduce the fraction.

Example 4

Change 3.055 into a fraction.

$$3.055 \rightarrow 3\frac{55}{1000} \rightarrow 3\frac{11}{200}$$

Steps

1. The 5 is located in the thousandths place.
2. The numerator becomes 55 and 1,000 becomes the denominator. The 3 is still the whole number.
3. Reduce the fraction.

Change the following decimals into fractions and reduce to the lowest common denominator.

1. 0.08 =
2. 0.025 =
3. 0.125 =
4. 0.17 =
5. 0.3 =
6. 2.75 =
7. 7.07 =
8. 12.0001 =
9. 3.48 =
10. 0.275 =

Ratios and Proportions

Vocabulary

Ratio: A relationship between two numbers.
Proportion: Two ratios that have equal values.

HESI Hint

Ratios can be written several ways.

As a fraction: $\frac{5}{12}$

Using a colon: 5:12
In words: 5 to 12

Proportions can be written two ways.

$$\frac{5}{12} = \frac{25}{60}$$

$$5:12::25:60$$

NOTE: The numerator is listed first, then the denominator.

Example 1

Change the decimal to a ratio.

$$0.025 \rightarrow \frac{25}{1000} \rightarrow \frac{1}{40} \rightarrow 1:40$$

Steps

1. Change the decimal to a fraction.
2. Reduce the fraction.
3. The numerator (1) is the first listed number.
4. Then write the colon.
5. Finally, place the denominator (40) after the colon.

Example 2

Change the fraction to a ratio.

$$\frac{5}{6} = 5:6$$

Steps

1. The numerator (5) is the first listed number.
2. Then write the colon.
3. Finally, place the denominator (6) after the colon.

Example 3

Solve the proportion (find the value of x).
7:10 :: 14:x

$$7:10 \ :: 14:x$$
$$\frac{7}{10} = \frac{14}{x}$$
$$\frac{7}{10} \overset{x2}{\underset{x2}{=}} \frac{14}{x}$$
$$\frac{7}{10} = \frac{14}{x}$$
$$x = 20$$

Steps

1. Rewrite the proportion as a fraction (this might help to see the solution).
2. Note that $7 \times 2 = 14$; therefore $10 \times 2 = 20$.
   - Multiply 14×10 (two diagonal numbers). The answer is 140.
   - $140 \div 7 = 20$ (Divide the remaining number.)
3. The answer is 20.

Example 4

Solve the proportion (find the value of x).
x:63 :: 24:72.

$$\frac{x}{63} = \frac{24}{72}$$
$$\frac{x}{63} = \frac{24}{72}$$
$$24 \times 63 = 1512$$
$$1,512 \div 72 = 21$$
$$x = 21$$

Steps

1. Rewrite the proportion as a fraction.
2. Multiply the diagonal numbers: $24 \times 63 = 1512$.
3. Divide the answer (1,512) by the remaining number: $1,512 \div 72 = 21$.
4. The value for x is 21.

Example 5

Solve the proportion (find the value of x).
240:60 :: x:12.

$$\frac{240}{60} = \frac{x}{12}$$
$$\frac{240}{60} = \frac{x}{12}$$
$$x = 48$$

Steps

1. Rewrite the proportion as a fraction.
2. Multiply the diagonal numbers together: $240 \times 12 = 2,880$.
3. Divide the answer (2,880) by the remaining number: $2,880 \div 60 = 48$.
4. The answer to x is 48.

Change the following fractions to ratios:

1. $\dfrac{22}{91}$

2. $\dfrac{19}{40}$

Solve the following for *x*:

3. 7:5 :: 91:*x*
4. 7:9 :: *x*:63
5. *x*:15 :: 120:225
6. 15:*x* :: 3:8
7. 360:60 :: 6:*x*
8. *x*:81 :: 9:27
9. John buys 3 bags of chips for $4.50. How much will it cost John to buy five bags of chips?
10. The recipe states that 4 cups of sugar will make 144 cookies. How many cups of sugar are needed to make 90 cookies?

Percentages

Vocabulary

Percent: Per hundred (part per hundred).

Example 1

Change the decimal to a **percent:** 0.13 → 13%.

Steps

1. Move the decimal point to the right of the hundredths place (two places).
2. Put the percent sign behind the new number.

Example 2

Change the decimal to a percent: 0.002 → 0.2%.

Steps

1. Move the decimal point to the right of the hundredths place (always two places!).
2. Put the percent sign behind the new number. It is still a percent; it is just a very small percent.

Example 3

Change the percent to a decimal: 85.4% → 0.854.

Steps

1. Move the decimal two spaces away from the percent sign (to the left).
2. Drop the percent sign; it is no longer a percent, but a decimal.

Example 4

Change the percent to a decimal: 75% → 0.75.

Steps

1. The decimal point is not visible but is always located after the last number.
2. Move the decimal two spaces away from the percent sign (toward the left).
3. Drop the percent sign; the number is no longer a percent, but a decimal.

Example 5

Change the fraction to a percent: $\dfrac{5}{6}$

$$
\begin{array}{r}
.833 \\
6\overline{)5.000} \\
-48\downarrow\downarrow \\
\hline
20\downarrow \\
-18\downarrow \\
\hline
20
\end{array}
$$

$0.833 \rightarrow 83.3\%$

Steps

1. Change the fraction into a division problem and solve.
2. Move the decimal behind the hundredths place in the quotient.
3. Place a percent sign after the new number.

SAMPLE PROBLEMS

Change the following decimals to percents.

1. $0.98 =$
2. $0.0068 =$
3. $0.09 =$

Change the following percents to decimals.

4. $58\% =$
5. $76.3\% =$
6. $0.03\% =$

Change the following fractions to percents.

7. $\dfrac{9}{10} =$

8. $\dfrac{4}{5} =$

9. $\dfrac{1}{6} =$

10. $\dfrac{3}{8} =$

Using the Percent Formula

HESI Hint

The word *of* usually indicates the whole portion of the percent formula.
Percent formula:

$$\frac{\text{Part}}{\text{Whole}} = \frac{\%}{100}$$

Using this formula will help in all percent problems in which there is an unknown (solving for *x*).

Example 1

What is 7 out of 8 expressed as a percent?

$$\frac{7}{8} = \frac{\%}{100}$$
$$7 \times 100 = 700$$
$$700 \div 8 = 87.5$$
$$\% = 87.5 \text{ or } 87.5\%$$

Steps

1. Rewrite the problem using the percent formula.
2. Multiply the diagonal numbers together: $7 \times 100 = 700$.
3. Divide by the remaining number: $700 \div 8 = 87.5\%$.

Example 2

What is 68% of 45?

$$\frac{x}{45} = \frac{68}{100}$$
$$45 \times 68 - 3,060$$
$$3,060 \div 100 = 30.6$$
$$x = 30.6$$

Steps

1. Rewrite the problem using the percent formula.
2. "Of 45:" 45 is the whole.
3. Multiply the diagonal numbers together: $68 \times 45 = 3,060$.
4. Divide by the remaining number: $3,060 \div 100 = 30.6$.
5. $x = 30.6$ (this is not a percent; it is the part).

Example 3

18 is 50% of what number?

$$\frac{18}{x} = \frac{50}{100}$$
$$18 \times 100 = 1,800$$
$$1,800 \div 50 = 36$$
$$x = 36$$

Steps

1. Rewrite the problem using the percent formula.
2. We are looking for the **whole** because *of* is indicating an unknown number.
3. Multiply the diagonal numbers together: $18 \times 100 = 1800$.
4. Divide by the remaining number: $1,800 \div 50 = 36$.

Fractions, Decimals, and Percents

Fraction	Decimal	Percent
$\frac{1}{2}$	0.50	50%
$\frac{1}{4}$	0.25	25%
$\frac{3}{4}$	0.75	75%
$\frac{1}{5}$	0.20	20%
$\frac{2}{5}$	0.40	40%
$\frac{3}{5}$	0.60	60%
$\frac{4}{5}$	0.80	80%
$\frac{1}{8}$	0.125	12.5%
$\frac{3}{8}$	0.375	37.5%
$\frac{5}{8}$	0.625	62.5%
$\frac{7}{8}$	0.875	87.5%
$\frac{1}{3}$	$0.33\bar{3}$	33.3%
$\frac{2}{3}$	$0.66\bar{6}$	66.6%

SAMPLE PROBLEMS

Solve the following percent problems.
1. What is 15 out of 75 as a percent?
2. What is 2 out of 50 as a percent?
3. What is 20 out of 100 as a percent?
4. What is 28% of 100?
5. What is 95% of 20?
6. What is 15.5% of 600?
7. The number 2 is 20% of what number?
8. The number 65 is 25% of what number?
9. The number 9 is 20% of what number?
10. The number 44 is 25% of what number?

Regular Time versus Military Time

Regular time uses the numbers 1 through 12 with the suffixes AM or PM to represent the hour in a 24-hour period. Military time uses the numbers 00 through 23 to represent the hour in a 24-hour period. The minutes and seconds in regular and military time are expressed the same way.

HESI Hint

To convert to military time before noon, simply include a zero before the numbers 1 through 9 for AM. For example, 9:35 AM regular time converts to 0935 military time. The zero is not needed when converting 10 AM or 11 AM. If the time is after noon, simply add 12 to the hour number. For example, 1:30 PM regular time converts to 1330 military time (1 + 12 = 13). Midnight, or 12 AM, is converted to 0000. Noon, or 12 PM, is converted to 1200.

Table 1-1 summarizes the equivalents between military time and regular time. Military time is written with a colon between the minutes and seconds just as in regular time. It can also be expressed with a colon between the hours and the minutes. Military time is written as follows:

hoursminutes:seconds	OR	**hours**:minutes:seconds
0932:24 hours	OR	**09**:23:24
1926:56 hours	OR	**19**:26:56 hours

Regular time is written as follows:

hours:minutes:seconds AM or PM
9:32:24 AM
7:26:56 PM

Table 1-1 Equivalents for Military Time and Regular Time

Military Time	Regular Time	Military Time	Regular Time
0000	12:00 AM (Midnight)	1200	12:00 PM (Noon)
0100	1:00 AM	1300	1:00 PM
0200	2:00 AM	1400	2:00 PM
0300	3:00 AM	1500	3:00 PM
0400	4:00 AM	1600	4:00 PM
0500	5:00 AM	1700	5:00 PM
0600	6:00 AM	1800	6:00 PM
0700	7:00 AM	1900	7:00 PM
0800	8:00 AM	2000	8:00 PM
0900	9:00 AM	2100	9:00 PM
1000	10:00 AM	2200	10:00 PM
1100	11:00 AM	2300	11:00 PM

SAMPLE PROBLEMS

Convert the following regular times to military times.
1. 12:00 AM =
2. 3:30 PM =

3. 11:19:46 AM =
4. 8:22:54 PM =
5. 4:27:33 PM =
6. 2:22:22 AM =

Convert the following military times to regular times.
7. 0603:45 hours
8. 1200:00 hours
9. 15:16:42 hours
10. 16:18:00 hours
11. 10:33:29 hours
12. 21:11:34 hours

Algebra

Vocabulary

Variable: A letter representing an unknown quantity (i.e., x).
Constant: A number that cannot change.
Expression: A mathematical sentence containing constants and variables (i.e., $3x - 2$).
Exponent: A number or symbol placed above and after another number or symbol (a superscript or subscript), indicating the number of times to multiply.

Algebra is a process that involves variables and constants. A **variable** is a letter that represents an unknown quantity. A **constant** is a number that cannot change. Using the operations of addition, subtraction, multiplication, and division, we can use algebra to find the value of unknown quantities. Two algebra concepts discussed in this section will be evaluating **expressions** and solving equations for a specific variable.

HESI Hint

When working with algebra, remember to evaluate expressions by performing the "Order of Operations:"

1. Evaluate numbers within parentheses.	$4 \cdot (2 + 3)^2 - 5$
2. Multiply numbers based on any exponents.	$4 \cdot (5)^2 - 5$
3. Multiply and divide numbers from left to right.	$4 \cdot 25 - 5$
4. Add and subtract numbers from left to right.	$100 - 5$

The variable for these expressions is 95.

Here's a mnemonic to remember the "Order of Operations":
"Please excuse my dear Aunt Sally" helps to remember the correct order of operations. The order should be Parentheses, Exponents, Multiply, Divide, Add, Subtract.

Evaluating the Expression

When we substitute a specific value for each variable in the expression and then perform the operations, it's called "evaluating the expression."

Example 1

Evaluate the expression $ab + c$ if $a = 4$, $b = -2$, and $c = 7$

$$(4)(-2) + (7)$$
$$-8 + 7$$
$$-1$$

Steps

1. Substitute the numbers into the given expression. Use parentheses when inserting numbers into an expression.
2. Multiply $4 \times -2 = -8$
3. Add $-8 + 7 = -1$

Example 2

Evaluate the expression $-xy(x - y) + y$ if $x = 4$ and $y = -2$

$$-(4)(-2)([4] - [-2]) + (-2)$$
$$-(-8)(4 + 2) - 2$$
$$8(6) - 2$$
$$48 - 2$$
$$46$$

Steps

1. Substitute the numbers into the given expression.
2. Multiply $4 \times -2 = -8$.
3. Change $-(-2)$ to $+2$, and $+(-2)$ to -2.
4. Add $4 + 2 = 6$
5. Change $-(-8)$ to 8
6. Multiply $8 \times 6 = 48$
7. Subtract $48 - 2 = 46$

Solving Equations for a Specific Variable

To solve equations for a specific variable, perform the operations in the reverse order in which you evaluate expressions.

Example 3

$$\text{Solve}: \quad 4x + 5 = 17$$
$$\underline{\quad -5 \quad -5}$$
$$\frac{4x}{4} = \frac{12}{4}$$
$$x = 3$$

Steps

1. Subtract 5 from each side of the equation.
2. Divide both sides by 4.

Example 4

$$\text{Solve}: \quad -7k - 4 = -21$$
$$\underline{\quad +4 = +4}$$
$$\frac{-7k}{-7} = \frac{-17}{-7}$$
$$k = \frac{17}{7}$$

Steps

1. Add 4 to both sides.
2. Divide both sides by -7.
3. Simplify. (A negative divided by a negative is a positive.)

Evaluate the following expressions:
1. $xm - 2m$ if $x = -2$ and $m = -3$
2. $2abc - 3ab$ if $a = 2, b = -3,$ and $c = 4$
3. $-x(y + z)$ if $x = 4, y = -3,$ and $z = -5$
4. $-k + h + kh$ if $k = -5$ and $h = -2$
5. $-(a - b)(a - bc)$ if $a = 3, b = -4,$ and $c = 2$

Solve the following equations for the given variable:
6. $3x - 5 = 10$ solve for x.
7. $-2x - 2 = 14$ solve for x.
8. $2y + 3 = 12$ solve for y.
9. $4x + 5 = -19$ solve for x.
10. $-5 = 6m - 1$ solve for m.

Helpful Information to Memorize

Roman Numerals

I = 1	XX = 20	M = 1,000
II = 2	XXX = 30	$\overline{V}$ = 5,000
III = 3	XL = 40	$\overline{X}$ = 10,000
IV = 4	L = 50	$\overline{L}$ = 50,000
V = 5	LX = 60	$\overline{C}$ = 100,000
VI = 6	LXX = 70	$\overline{D}$ = 500,000
VII = 7	LXXX = 80	$\overline{M}$ = 1,000,000
VIII = 8	XC = 90	
IX = 9	C = 100	
X = 10	D = 500	
XI = 11		
Example 2012 = MMXII		

Measurement Conversions

TEMPERATURE	
0° Celsius = 32° Fahrenheit (the freezing point of water)	
100° Celsius = 212° Fahrenheit (the boiling point of water)	
LENGTH	
Metric	**English**
1 kilometer = 1,000 meters	1 mile = 1,760 yards
1 meter = 100 centimeters	1 mile = 5,280 feet
1 centimeter = 10 millimeters	1 yard = 3 feet
2.54 centimeters = 1 inch	1 foot = 12 inches
VOLUME AND CAPACITY	
Metric	**English**
1 liter = 1,000 milliliters	1 gallon = 4 quarts
1 milliliter = 1 cubic centimeter	1 gallon = 128 ounces
	1 quart = 2 pints
	1 pint = 2 cups
	1 cup = 8 ounces
	1 ounce = 30 milliliters (cubic centimeters)
WEIGHT AND MASS	
Metric	**English**
1 kilogram = 1,000 grams	1 ton = 2,000 pounds
1 gram = 1,000 milligrams	1 pound = 16 ounces
	2.2 pounds = 1 kilogram

Answers to Sample Problems

Basic Addition and Subtraction

1. 1,959
2. 980
3. 1,511
4. 200
5. 432
6. 459
7. 108
8. 12,011
9. 13 miles
10. 19

Basic Multiplication (Whole Numbers)

1. 5,922
2. 1,950
3. 7,836

4. 44,330
5. 11,130
6. 21,978
7. 189,150
8. 1,557,270
9. 870
10. 180

Basic Division (Whole Numbers)

1. 12
2. 3,206
3. 1,233
4. 25
5. 628
6. 741
7. 214.75
8. 998.14
9. 9
10. 11

Addition and Subtraction of Decimals

1. 16.75
2. 66.838
3. 948.2
4. 25.26
5. 30.05
6. 10.45
7. 29.41
8. 12.57
9. 3.75
10. 2.5

Multiplication of Decimals

1. 0.01269
2. 786.08
3. 16.863
4. 6252.5
5. 0.287804
6. 32.92
7. 3.7236
8. 0.79423
9. 19.2
10. 4.375

Division of Decimals

1. 120
2. 240
3. 9.375

4. 281
5. 8.23
6. 1,970
7. 0.9
8. 1.2
9. 224
10. 6

Addition of Fractions

1. $\dfrac{1}{2}$

2. $\dfrac{17}{21}$

3. $1\dfrac{3}{10}$

4. $\dfrac{13}{14}$

5. $1\dfrac{23}{35}$

6. $9\dfrac{11}{24}$

7. $6\dfrac{4}{9}$

8. $15\dfrac{8}{21}$

9. $4\dfrac{1}{6}$

10. $25\dfrac{5}{8}$

Subtraction of Fractions

1. $\dfrac{1}{20}$

2. $\dfrac{11}{37}$

3. $\dfrac{2}{25}$

4. $\dfrac{1}{54}$

5. $1\dfrac{7}{10}$

6. $15\dfrac{1}{18}$

7. $12\dfrac{3}{7}$

8. $16\dfrac{3}{4}$

9. $1\dfrac{3}{8}$ feet

10. $\dfrac{11}{12}$ cups

Multiplication of Fractions

1. $\dfrac{2}{5}$

2. $\dfrac{7}{81}$

3. $4\dfrac{4}{5}$

4. 7

5. $3\dfrac{3}{4}$

6. 8

7. $6\dfrac{2}{3}$

8. $7\dfrac{1}{2}$

9. $16\dfrac{1}{2}$

10. $27\dfrac{13}{16}$

Division of Fractions

1. $5\dfrac{3}{5}$

2. $1\dfrac{1}{3}$

3. $5\dfrac{1}{4}$

4. 5

5. 32

6. 9

7. 3

8. $6\dfrac{1}{6}$

9. 15

10. 10

Changing Fractions to Decimals

1. 0.2
2. 0.4
3. 0.375

4. 0.8
5. 0.333
6. 1.5
7. 0.3
8. 2.875
9. 11.733
10. 0.44

Changing Decimals to Fractions

1. $\dfrac{2}{25}$

2. $\dfrac{1}{40}$

3. $\dfrac{1}{8}$

4. $\dfrac{17}{100}$

5. $\dfrac{3}{10}$

6. $2\dfrac{3}{4}$

7. $7\dfrac{7}{100}$

8. $12\dfrac{1}{10000}$

9. $3\dfrac{12}{25}$

10. $\dfrac{11}{40}$

Ratios and Proportions

1. 22:91
2. 19:40
3. $x = 65$
4. $x = 49$
5. $x = 8$
6. $x = 40$
7. $x = 1$
8. $x = 27$
9. $x = \$7.50$
10. $x = 2.5$

Percentages

1. 98%
2. 0.68%
3. 9%
4. 0.58

5. 0.763
6. 0.0003
7. 90%
8. 80%
9. 16.667%
10. 37.5%

Using the Percent Formula

1. 20%
2. 4%
3. 20%
4. 28
5. 19
6. 93
7. 10
8. 260
9. 45
10. 176

Regular Time versus Military Time

1. 0000 hours OR 00:00 hours
2. 1530 hours OR 15:30 hours
3. 1119:46 hours OR 11:19:46 hours
4. 2022:54 hours OR 20:22:54 hours
5. 1627:33 hours OR 16:27:33 hours
6. 0222:22 hours OR 02:22:22 hours
7. 6:03:45 AM
8. 12:00 PM OR Noon
9. 3:16:42 PM
10. 4:18 PM
11. 10:33:29 AM
12. 9:11:34 PM

Algebra

1. 12
2. −30
3. 32
4. 13
5. −77
6. $x = 5$
7. $x = -8$
8. $y = \dfrac{9}{2}$ or $y = 4\dfrac{1}{2}$ or $y = 4.5$
9. $x = -6$
10. $m = -\dfrac{2}{3}$

2 READING COMPREHENSION

C ommunication, whether written or spoken, sets us apart from all other life forms. We live in an age of instant telecommunication and think nothing of it. Yet, it is the written word that allows a person to record information that can travel across time and distance, to be examined and reexamined. In the health care setting, this is especially true for the health care provider. The client record is written documentation of what is known of the client, which includes health care history, the evaluation or assessment, the diagnosis, the treatment, the care, the progress, and possibly, the outcome. A clear understanding of all client information ensures better health care management for the client. The ability to skillfully read and understand also helps the health care provider clearly document the client's written record as care is provided. Any student wishing to enter the health care profession must have the ability to read and understand the written word.

CHAPTER OUTLINE

Identifying the Main Idea
Identifying Supporting Details
Finding the Meaning of Words in
   Context

Identifying a Writer's Purpose
   and Tone
Distinguishing between
   Fact and Opinion

Making Logical Inferences
Summarizing
Review Questions
Answers to Review Questions

KEY TERMS

Antonym
Assumption
Connotation

Context Clue
Inference

Synonym
Tone

Identifying the Main Idea

Identifying the main idea is the key to understanding what has been read and what needs to be remembered. First, identify the topic of the passage or paragraph by asking the question, "What is it about?" Once that question has been answered, ask, "What point is the author making about the topic?" If the reader understands the author's message about the topic, then the main idea has been identified.

In longer passages the reader might find it helpful to count the number of paragraphs used to describe what is believed to be the main idea statement. If the majority of paragraphs include information about the main idea statement the reader has chosen, then the reader is probably correct. However, if the answer chosen by the reader is mentioned in only one paragraph, then the main idea that was chosen is probably just a detail.

Another helpful hint in identifying main ideas is to read a paragraph and then stop and summarize that paragraph. This type of active reading helps the reader focus on the content and can lessen the need to reread the entire passage several times.

Some students find that visualizing as they read helps them remember details and stay focused. They picture the information they are reading as if it were being projected on a big-screen TV. If you do not already do this, try it. Informal classroom experiments have proved that students who visualize while reading comprehension tests easily outscore their counterparts who do not visualize.

HESI Hint

Main ideas can be found in the beginning, in the middle, or at the end of a paragraph or passage. Always check the introduction and conclusion for the main idea.

Finally, not all main ideas are stated. Identify unstated or implied main ideas by looking specifically at the details, examples, causes, and reasons given.

Again, asking the questions stated earlier will help in this task:

- What is the passage about? (Topic)
- What point is the author making about the topic? (Main idea)

Some experts like to compare the main idea with an umbrella covering all or most of the details in a paragraph or passage. The chosen main idea can be tested for accuracy by asking whether the other details will fit under the umbrella. The idea of an umbrella also helps visualize how broad a statement the main idea can be.

Identifying Supporting Details

Writing is made up of main ideas and details. Few would enjoy reading only a writer's main ideas. The details provide the interest, the visual picture, and the examples that sustain a reader's interest.

Often students confuse the author's main idea with the examples or reasons the author gives to support the main idea. These details give the reader a description, the background, or simply more information to support the writer's assertion or main idea. Without these details, the reader would not be able to evaluate whether the writer has made his or her case nor would the reader find the passage as interesting. In addition to examples, facts and statistics may be used.

The reader's job is to distinguish between the details, which support the writer's main idea, and the main idea itself. Usually the reader can discover clues to help identify details because often an author uses transition words such as *one, next, another, first,* or *finally* to indicate that a detail is being provided.

Finding the Meaning of Words in Context

Even the most avid of readers will come across words for which they do not know the meaning. Identifying the correct meanings of these words may be the key to identifying the author's main idea and to fully comprehending the author's meaning. The reader can, of course, stop and use a dictionary for these words. However, this is usually neither the most efficient nor the most practical way to approach these unknown words.

There are other options the reader can use to find the meanings of unknown words, and these involve using context clues. The phrase **context clue** refers to the information provided by the author in the words or sentences surrounding the unknown word or words.

Some of the easiest context clues to recognize are as follows:

1. Definition—The author puts the meaning of the word in parentheses or states the definition in the following sentence.

2. **Synonym**—The author gives the reader another word that means the same or nearly the same as the unknown word.

3. **Antonym**—The author gives a word that means the opposite of the unknown word.

HESI Hint

The reader needs to watch for clue words such as *although, but,* and *instead,* which sometimes signal that an antonym is being used.

4. Restatement—The author restates the unknown word in a sentence using more familiar words.

5. Examples—The author gives examples that clearly help the reader understand the meaning of the unknown word.

6. Explanation—The author gives more information about the unknown word, which better explains the meaning of the word.

7. Word structure—Sometimes simply knowing the meanings of basic prefixes, suffixes, and root words can help the reader make an educated guess about an unknown word.

HESI Hint

When being tested on finding the meaning of a word in the context of a passage, look carefully at the words and sentences surrounding the unknown word. The context clues are usually there for the reader to uncover. Once the correct meaning has been chosen, test that meaning in the passage. It should make sense, and the meaning should be supported by the other sentences in the passage or paragraph.

Identifying a Writer's Purpose and Tone

The purposes or reasons for reading or writing are similar for the readers and the writers. Readers read to be entertained, and authors write to entertain. Readers choose to read for information, and writers write to inform. However, in the area of persuasion, a reader can be fooled into believing he/she is reading something objective when in fact the author is trying to manipulate the reader's thinking, which is why it is important for readers to ask the following questions:

1. Who is the intended audience?
2. Why is this being written?

If the writer is trying to change the reader's thinking, encourage the reader to buy something, or convince the reader to vote for someone, the reader can assume the writer's goal is to persuade. More evidence can be found to determine the writer's purpose by identifying specific words used within the passage. Words that are biased, or words that have positive or negative connotations, will often help the reader determine the author's reason for writing. (**Connotation** refers to the emotions or feelings that the reader attaches to words.)

If the writer uses a number of words with negative or positive connotations, the writer is usually trying to manipulate the reader's thinking about a person, place, or thing. Looking at the writer's choice of words also helps the reader determine the tone of the passage. (An author's **tone** refers to the attitude or feelings the author has about the topic.)

For example, if the author is writing about the Dallas City Council's decision to build waterways on the Trinity River bottom to resemble the San Antonio River Walk and describes this decision as being "inspired" and "visionary," the reader knows the author has positive feelings about the decision. The tone of this article is positive because the words *inspired* and *visionary* are positive words. The reader might also be aware that the author may be trying to manipulate the reader's thinking.

On the other hand, if the writer describes the council's decision as being "wasteful" and "foolhardy," the reader knows the author has negative feelings about the council's decision. The reader can determine that the tone is unfavorable because of the words the writer chose. Typically, articles with obvious positive or negative tones and connotations will be found on the opinion or editorial page of the newspaper.

Articles or books written to inform should be less biased, and information should be presented in factual format and with sufficient supporting data to allow readers to form their own opinions on the event that occurred.

HESI Hint

When determining the writer's purpose and/or tone, look closely at the writer's choice of words. The words are the key clues.

Distinguishing between Fact and Opinion

A critical reader must be an active reader. A critical reader must question and evaluate the writer's underlying assumptions. An **assumption** is a set of beliefs that the writer has about the subject. A critical reader must determine whether the writer's statements are facts or opinions and whether the supporting evidence and details are relevant and valid. A critical reader is expected to determine whether the author's argument is credible and logical.

To distinguish between fact and opinion, the reader must understand the common definitions of those words. A fact is considered something that can be proved (either right or wrong). For example, at the time Columbus sailed for the New World, it was considered a scientific fact that the world was flat. Columbus proved the scientists wrong.

An opinion is a statement that cannot be proved. For example, "I thought the movie *Avatar* was the best movie ever made" is a statement of opinion. It is subjective; it is the writer's personal opinion. On the other hand, the following is a statement of fact: "The movie *Avatar* was nominated for an Academy Award for best picture in 2010 but did not win." This statement is a fact because it can be proved to be correct.

Again, the reader must look closely at the writer's choice of words in determining fact or opinion. Word choices that include measurable data and colors are considered factual or concrete words. "Frank weighs 220 pounds" and "Mary's dress is red" are examples of concrete words being used in statements of fact.

If the writer uses evaluative or judgmental words (*good, better, best, worst*), it is considered a statement of opinion. Abstract words (*love, hate, envy*) are also used in statements of opinion. These include ideas or concepts that cannot be measured. Statements that deal with probabilities or speculations about future events are also considered opinions.

Making Logical Inferences

In addition to determining fact and opinion, a critical reader is constantly required to make logical inferences. An **inference** is an educated guess or conclusion drawn by the reader based on the available facts and information. Although this may sound difficult and sometimes is, it is done all the time. A critical reader does not always know whether the inference is correct, but the inference is made based on the reader's own set of beliefs or assumptions.

Determining inferences is a skill often referred to as *reading between the lines*. It is a logical connection that is based on the situation, the facts provided, and the reader's knowledge and experience. The key to making logical inferences is to be sure the inferences are supportable by evidence or facts presented in the reading. This often requires reading the passage twice so that details can be identified. Inferences are not stated in the reading but are derived from the information presented and influenced by the reader's knowledge and experience.

Summarizing

Identifying the best summary of a reading selection is a skill most students find frustrating. Yet this skill can be mastered easily when the following three rules are used:

1. The summary should include the main ideas from the beginning, middle, and end of the passage.
2. The summary must be presented in sequence; it cannot move from the beginning to the end and then back to the middle.
3. The summary must have accurate information. Sometimes a test summary will deliberately include false information. In that case, the critical reader will automatically throw that test option out.

This type of question will typically take the longest for the student to answer, because to answer it correctly the student must go through each summary choice and locate the related information or main idea in the passage itself. Double-checking the summary choices is one way of proving that the reader has the best summary, because if the summary choice presents information that is inaccurate or out of order, the reader will automatically eliminate those choices.

HESI Hint

Remember, the summary should include the main ideas of the passage, possibly with some major supporting details. Finally, it is a shortened version of the passage that includes all the important information, eliminating the unnecessary and redundant.

REVIEW QUESTIONS

Each year, more and more "baby boomers" reach the age of 65 and become eligible for Medicare. As of July 2009, according to the Census Bureau, approximately 13% of the population in the United States is 65 years of age or older. It is projected that this group will increase to 21% of the population by 2050. As health care costs go up and needs increase with age, Medicare is especially important to seniors. Medicare Part A provides assistance with inpatient hospital costs, whereas Part B helps pay for doctor services and outpatient care. In 2006, Congress enacted Medicare Part D, which today helps many seniors pay for the cost of prescription drugs.

Before the enactment of Medicare Part D, many seniors faced financial hardship in regards to prescription drugs. Today, it is no longer a question of housing costs and food versus prescription drugs, but which Part D plan provides the best coverage. Although Part D has alleviated many uncertainties, there are still concerns. Not all prescription drugs are covered in each plan provided by Part D. Each plan has its own list of covered drugs that can change at any time, requiring seniors to possibly switch coverage every year. Seniors who suffer from multiple medical conditions may not be able to find a plan that covers all prescribed medication. In addition to a monthly premium paid for Part D, once prescription costs reach $2830, the participant is responsible for all drug costs up to $4450. This "donut hole," as it is known, can mean that some seniors reduce or stop their medication for the remainder of the program year.

Medicare helps provide seniors with some of the best health care in the world. Yet, it does come at a huge financial cost that might behoove younger generations to consider preventive care to improve those golden years.

1. What is the main idea of the passage?
   A. The high cost of prescription drugs is a difficult financial burden for seniors.
   B. Medicare Part D has many problems and no benefits.
   C. Medicare Part D, along with Part A and Part B, helps seniors afford prescription drugs and better health care.
   D. Senior citizens enrolled in Medicare Part D have no prescription drug concerns.

2. Which of the following is not listed as a detail in the passage?
   A. By the year 2050 the number of seniors over the age of 65 will increase.
   B. Medicare Parts A and B help pay for hospital costs and doctor services.
   C. Seniors are required to enroll in Medicare Part D.
   D. Medicare Part D includes a "donut hole."

3. What is the meaning of the word *behoove* as used in the last paragraph?
   A. To be needful
   B. To be responsible for
   C. To increase
   D. To tell others

4. What is the author's primary purpose in writing this essay?
   A. To inform people how to enroll in Medicare
   B. To persuade seniors to enroll in Medicare Part D
   C. To entertain non–health care professionals
   D. To analyze the provisions of Medicare Part D

5. Identify the overall tone of the essay.
   A. Argumentative
   B. Cautious
   C. Sympathetic
   D. Pessimistic

6. Which of the following statements is an opinion?
   A. Senior citizens pay a monthly insurance premium for Part D coverage.
   B. The high cost of prescription drugs has made life difficult for seniors.
   C. In 2006, Congress enacted Medicare legislation that provides prescription drug coverage.
   D. Not all prescription drugs are covered in each plan provided by Medicare Part D.

7. Which statement would not be inferred by the reader?
   A. Most Americans will never have a need for Medicare and its various parts.
   B. Some age-related illnesses might be averted with preventive care.
   C. Some seniors could find themselves changing their Part D coverage yearly.

D. The "donut hole" in Part D does create a financial hardship for seniors.

8. Choose the best summary of the passage.

A. Americans are growing older every year and are requiring more and more health care. Health care professionals can help meet those needs if seniors enroll in Medicare Parts A, B, and D. The three parts of Medicare can ease the financial burden of seniors.

B. At the age of 65, senior citizens sign up for Medicare Parts A, B, and D that will cover medical costs up to $2830 a year. For those seniors who suffer from multiple health issues the cost is $4450. Prescription drug care provided through Part D makes life much easier for seniors.

C. "Baby boomers" are the most common senior citizens requiring health care. This group is the fastest growing group and will comprise 21% of the population by 2050. Even though there are concerns about Medicare, Part D ensures that all seniors have the medical coverage they need.

D. Medicare Parts A, B, and D help seniors pay for hospital costs, doctor and outpatient services, and most recently, prescription drugs. Even though Part D offers many benefits, concerns about various plans with different covered prescriptions and the "donut hole" are still of concern. For seniors, life with Medicare is much better.

ANSWERS TO REVIEW QUESTIONS

1. C—main idea
2. C—supporting detail
3. A—meaning of word in context
4. D—author's purpose
5. B—author's tone
6. B—fact and opinion
7. A—inferences
8. D—summary

Bibliography

Johnson B: *The reading edge,* ed 4, New York, 2001, Houghton Mifflin.

3 VOCABULARY

Members of the health professions use specific medical terminology to ensure accurate, concise, and consistent communication among all persons involved in the provision of health care. In addition to the use of specific medical terms, many general vocabulary words are used in a health care context. It is essential that students planning to enter the health care field have a basic understanding of these general vocabulary words to ensure accurate communication in a professional setting.

The following list of vocabulary words includes a definition for each word and an example of the word as used in a health care context. Careful study and review of these vocabulary words will help you begin your health profession studies with the ability to communicate in a professional manner.

HESI Hint

Being able to use a wide range of vocabulary skills correctly is considered by some experts to be the best measure of adult IQ.

Abrupt: Sudden.

Example: The nurse noticed an abrupt change in the patient's level of pain.

Abstain: To voluntarily refrain from something.

Example: The dental hygienist instructed the patient to abstain from smoking to improve his breath odor.

Access: A means to obtain entry or a means of approach.

Example: To administer medications into the patient's vein, the nurse must access the vein with a special needle.

Accountable: Responsible.

Example: Paramedics are accountable for maintaining up-to-date knowledge of resuscitation techniques.

Adhere: To hold fast or stick together.

Example: The tape must adhere to the patient's skin to hold the bandage in place.

Adverse: Undesired, possibly harmful.

Example: Vomiting is an adverse effect of many medications.

Affect: Appearance of observable emotions.

Example: The nurse observed that a depressed patient exhibited no obvious emotion and reported that the patient had a flat affect.

Annual: Occurring every year.

Example: The patient told the nurse that she had scheduled her annual mammogram, as she had been instructed.

Apply: To place, put on, or spread something.

Example: The physical therapist will apply a medication to the wound before covering the wound with a bandage.

Audible: Able to be heard.

Example: The respiratory therapist noticed that when the patient was having difficulty breathing, the therapist could hear an audible wheezing sound.

Bilateral: Present on two sides.

Example: The unlicensed assistive personnel reported to the nurse that the patient had bilateral weakness in the legs when walking.

Cardiac: Of or relating to the heart.

Example: Smoking increases the risk of cardiac disease.

Cast: Hard protective device applied to protect a broken bone while the bone heals.

Example: The nurse instructed the child that he could not go swimming while the cast was on his broken arm.

Cavity: An opening or an empty area.

Example: The nurse inspected the patient's oral cavity for lesions.

Cease: Come to an end or bring to an end.

Example: Because the patient's breathing had ceased, the paramedic began resuscitation measures.

Compensatory: Offsetting or making up for something.

Example: When the patient's blood pressure decreased, the paramedic noted that the heart rate increased, which the paramedic recognized as a compensatory action.

Complication: An undesired problem that is the result of some other event.

Example: The physician told the patient that loss of eyesight is a possible complication of eye surgery.

Comply: Do as directed.

Example: The nurse asked the patient to comply with the instructions for taking the medication.

Concave: Rounded inward.

Example: The dietician noticed that the patient was very thin and the patient's abdomen appeared concave.

Concise: Brief, to the point.

Example: When teaching a patient, the nurse tried to be concise, so the instructions would be easy to remember.

Consistency: Degree of viscosity; how thick or thin a fluid is.

Example: The respiratory therapist noticed that the mucus the patient was coughing was of a thin, watery consistency.

Constrict: To draw together or become smaller.

Example: The nurse knows that the small blood vessels of the skin will constrict when ice is applied to the skin.

Contingent: Dependent.

Example: The hygienist told the patient that a healthy mouth is contingent on careful daily brushing and flossing.

Contour: Shape or outline of a shape.

Example: While bathing an overweight patient, the unlicensed assistive personnel noticed that the contour of the patient's abdomen was quite rounded.

Contract: To draw together, to reduce in size.

Example: The physical therapist exercises the patient's muscles so they contract and expand.

Contraindication: A reason why something is not advisable or why it should not be done.

Example: The patient's excessive bleeding was a contraindication for discharge from the hospital.

Defecate: Expel feces.

Example: The unlicensed assistive personnel helped the patient to the toilet when he needed to defecate.

Deficit: A deficiency or lack of something.

Example: The therapist explained that the patient will experience a fluid deficit if the patient continues to perspire heavily during exercise without drinking enough fluids.

Depress: Press downward.

Example: The nurse will depress the patient's skin to see if any swelling is present.

Depth: Downward measurement from a surface.

Example: The physician measures the depth of a wound by inserting a cotton swab into the wound.

Deteriorating: Worsening.

Example: The dental hygienist explains that the condition of the patient's gums is deteriorating and treatment by the dentist is needed right away.

Device: Tool or piece of equipment.

Example: A thermometer is a device used to measure the patient's body temperature.

Diagnosis: Identification of an injury or disease.

Example: The patient received a diagnosis of pancreatitis.

Diameter: The distance across the center of an object.

Example: When measuring a patient's blood pressure, the nurse knows that when the diameter of a blood vessel increases, the pressure in that blood vessel goes down.

Dilate: To enlarge or expand.

Example: When shining a light in the patient's eyes, the nurse looks to see if both pupils dilate in response to the light.

Dilute: To make a liquid less concentrated.

Example: The nurse uses fruit juice to dilute a foul-tasting drug so that the medication will be easier to swallow.

Discrete: Distinct, separate.

Example: The paramedic observed several discrete bruise marks on the patient's body.

Distended: Enlarged or expanded from pressure.

Example: When a blood vessel is distended, the laboratory technician can easily insert a needle to obtain a blood sample.

Dysfunction: Impaired or abnormal functioning.

Example: Family dysfunction may increase when a member experiences an acute physical illness.

Elevate: To lift up or place in a higher position.

Example: The paramedic decided to elevate the head of the stretcher to help the patient breathe more easily.

Endogenous: Produced within the body.

Example: The nurse explained that endogenous insulin produced by the body's pancreas helps regulate the body's blood sugar levels.

Exacerbate: To make worse or more severe.

Example: The physical therapist recognized that too much exercise would exacerbate the patient's breathing difficulties.

Excess: More than what is needed or usual.

Example: The dietician explained that an excess consumption of caffeine may cause unpleasant effects such as feeling nervous and on edge.

Exogenous: Produced outside the body.

Example: The nurse explained that people with diabetes often need to receive exogenous forms of insulin because their bodies are unable to produce enough insulin.

Expand: To increase in size or amount.

Example: The unlicensed assistive personnel turns the patient frequently so that the size of the skin sore will not expand any further.

Exposure: Contact.

Example: The nurse taught the parents of a newborn to avoid exposure to people with severe infections.

External: Located outside the body.

Example: The unlicensed assistive personnel measured the amount of blood in the external drain after the patient's surgery.

Fatal: Resulting in death.

Example: The emergency medical technicians arrived too late to save any lives at the scene of a fatal car accident.

Fatigue: Extreme tiredness, exhaustion.

Example: The dietician explained to the patient that eating more iron-rich foods may help reduce feelings of fatigue.

Flaccid: Limp, lacking tone.

Example: After her stroke, the patient could not feed herself because her arms were flaccid.

Flushed: Reddened or ruddy appearance.

Example: The therapist observed that the patient's face was flushed after the patient completed the exercises.

Gaping: Wide open.

Example: In the emergency room, the nurse observed a gaping wound when examining a gunshot victim.

Gastrointestinal: Of or relating to the stomach and the intestines.

Example: The patient was diagnosed with a gastrointestinal disease.

Gender: Sex of an individual, as in male or female.

Example: Female gender places patients at higher risk for breast cancer.

Hematologic: Of or relating to blood.

Example: Pregnancy can put a woman at risk for anemia, which is a hematologic disorder

Hydration: Maintenance of body fluid balance.

Example: The nurse explains that adequate hydration helps keep skin soft and supple.

Hygiene: Measures contributing to cleanliness and good health.

Example: The dental assistant teaches patients about good hygiene practices to maintain strong teeth.

Impaired: Diminished or lacking some usual quality or level.

Example: The paramedic stated that the patient's impaired speech was obvious in the way she slurred her words.

Impending: Likely to occur soon.

Example: The nurse observed the patient signing the consent form for the impending procedure.

Incidence: Occurrence.

Example: In recent years there has been an increased incidence of infections that do not respond to antibiotics.

Infection: Contamination or invasion of body tissue by pathogenic organisms.

Example: The doctor prescribed antibiotics for the patient with a bacterial infection.

Inflamed: Reddened, swollen, warm, and often tender.

Example: The nurse observed that the skin around the patient's wound was inflamed.

Ingest: To swallow for digestion.

Example: The paramedic may contact the poison control center when providing emergency care for a child who has ingested cleaning fluid.

Initiate: To begin or put into practice.

Example: The nurse decided to initiate safety measures to prevent injury because the patient was very weak.

Insidious: So gradual as to not become apparent for a long time.

Example: The physician explained that the cancer probably started years ago but had not been detected because its spread was so insidious.

Intact: In place, unharmed.

Example: The nurse observed that the bandage was intact after surgery.

Internal: Located within the body.

Example: The paramedic reported that the patient was unconscious because of internal bleeding.

Invasive: Inserting or entering into a body part.

Example: The laboratory technician is careful when obtaining blood samples because this invasive procedure may cause problems such as infection or bruising.

Labile: Changing rapidly and often.

Example: Because the child's temperature was very labile, the nurse instructed the unlicensed assistive personnel to check the temperature frequently.

Laceration: Cut; tear.

Example: After the accident, the paramedic examined the patient's lacerations.

Latent: Present but not active or visible.

Example: The latent infection produced symptoms only when the patient's condition was weakened from another illness.

Lethargic: Difficult to arouse.

Example: The unlicensed assistive personnel observed that the morning after a patient received a sleeping pill, the patient was too lethargic to eat breakfast.

Manifestation: An indication or sign of a condition.

Example: The dietician looked for manifestations of poor nutrition, such as excessive weight loss and poor skin condition.

Musculoskeletal: Of or relating to muscle and skeleton.

Example: As a result of overtraining, the athlete suffered a musculoskeletal injury.

Neurologic: Of or relating to the nervous system.

Example: The nurse checked the neurologic status of the patient who was brought to the emergency room after a motorcycle accident.

Neurovascular: Of or relating to the nervous system and blood vessels.

Example: Strokes and aneurysms are neurovascular disorders.

Nutrient: Substance or ingredient that provides nourishment.

Example: The dietician explains that fruits and vegetables contain nutrients that reduce the risk of some cancers.

Occluded: Closed or obstructed.

Example: Because the patient's foot was cold and blue, the nurse reported that the patient's circulation to that foot was occluded.

Ominous: Significantly important and dangerous.

Example: After a patient sustained a head injury, the paramedic noted that the patient's breathing was irregular, which was an ominous sign that the patient's condition was worsening.

Ongoing: Continuous.

Example: The nurse instructed the patient that the treatment would be ongoing throughout the patient's entire hospital stay.

Oral: Given through or affecting the mouth.

Example: The unlicensed assistive personnel reminded the patient not to take any fluids orally because he is scheduled for surgery.

Overt: Obvious, easily observed.

Example: The overt symptoms of the disease included vomiting and diarrhea.

Parameter: A characteristic or constant factor, limit.

Example: The dietician explained that the number of calories needed for energy is one of the important parameters of a healthy diet.

Paroxysmal: Beginning suddenly or abruptly; convulsive.

Example: The respiratory therapist provided a breathing treatment to stop the patient's paroxysmal breathing difficulty.

Patent: Open.

Example: The nurse checked to see whether the intravenous needle was patent before giving the patient a medication.

Pathogenic: Causing or able to cause disease.

Example: Viruses and bacteria are pathogenic organisms.

Pathology: Processes, causes, and effects of a disease; abnormality.

Example: The doctor called to request the pathology report for her patient.

Posterior: Located behind; in the back.

Example: The dentist examined the posterior surface of the tooth for a cavity.

Potent: Producing a strong effect.

Example: The medication was very potent, and it immediately relieved the patient's pain.

Potential: Capable of occurring or likely to occur.

Example: Because the patient was very weak, the therapist felt the patient had a high potential for falling.

Precaution: Preventive measure.

Example: The laboratory technician wore gloves as a precaution against blood contamination.

Precipitous: Rapid, uncontrolled.

Example: The paramedic assisted the pregnant woman during a precipitous delivery in her home.

Predispose: To make more susceptible or more likely to occur.

Example: The dietician explains that high dietary fat intake predisposes some people to heart disease.

Preexisting: Already present.

Example: The nurse notified the physician that the patient has a preexisting condition that might lead to complications during the emergency surgery.

Primary: First or most significant.

Example: The patient's primary concern was when he could return to work after the operation.

Priority: Of great importance.

Example: The laboratory technician was gentle when inserting the needle because it is a high priority to ensure that the patient does not experience excessive pain and discomfort during the procedure.

Prognosis: The anticipated or expected course or outcome.

Example: The physician explained that with treatment the patient's prognosis was for a long and healthy life.

Rationale: The underlying reason.

Example: To make sure that the patient will follow the diet instructions, the dietician explains the rationale for the low-salt diet.

Recur: To occur again.

Example: To make sure that a tooth cavity does not recur, the dental hygienist instructs the patient to use toothpaste with fluoride regularly.

Renal: Of or relating to the kidneys.

Example: The nurse closely monitored the oral intake and urinary output of the patient with acute renal failure.

Respiration: Inhalation and exhalation of air.

Example: Exercise increases the rate and depth of an individual's respirations.

Restrict: To limit.

Example: The unlicensed assistive personnel removed the water pitcher from the room to assist the patient in following instructions to restrict the intake of fluids.

Retain: To hold or keep.

Example: The nurse administered a medication to prevent the patient from retaining excess body fluid, which might cause swelling.

Site: Location.

Example: The nurse selected a site to start the patient's IV based on the patient's comfort.

Status: Condition.

Example: The paramedic recognized that the patient's status was unstable, which necessitated immediate transport to the nearest medical center.

Strict: Stringent, exact, complete.

Example: The nurse stressed that the patient must follow instructions to maintain strict bed rest to prevent further injury.

Sublingual: Under the tongue.

Example: The patient was prescribed a sublingual medication for chest pain.

Supplement: To take in addition to or to complete.

Example: The dietician instructed the patients to supplement their diet with extra calcium tablets to help build strong bones.

Suppress: To stop or subdue.

Example: When the child's fever came down, the nurse checked to see if any medications had been given that would have suppressed the fever.

Symmetric (symmetrical): Being equal or the same in size, shape, and relative position.

Example: The paramedic observed that the movement of both sides of the patient's chest was symmetrical after the accident.

Symptom: An indication of a problem.

Example: The nurse recognized that the patient's weakness was a symptom of bleeding after surgery.

Syndrome: Group of symptoms that, when occurring together, reflect a specific disease or disorder.

Example: After reviewing the patient's symptoms, which included pain and tingling in the hand and fingers, the physician made a diagnosis of carpal tunnel syndrome.

Therapeutic: Of or relating to the treatment of a disease or a disorder.

Example: Therapeutic diets may include calorie and salt restrictions.

Transdermal: Crossing through the skin.

Example: The physician prescribed a transdermal nicotine patch for a patient participating in the smoking cessation program.

Transmission: Transfer, such as of a disease, from one person to another.

Example: Nurses should wash their hands to prevent the transmission of infections.

Trauma: Injury, wound.

Example: The accident victim had severe facial trauma.

Triage: Process used to determine the priority of treatment for patients according to the severity of a patient's condition and likelihood of benefit from the treatment.

Example: When the paramedics arrived at the scene of the accident, they had to triage the patients.

Untoward: Adverse or negative.

Example: The patient became very confused, which was an untoward effect of the medication received.

Urinate: Excrete or expel urine.

Example: The nurse instructed the patient to report any discomfort felt during urination.

Vascular: Of or relating to blood vessels.

Example: The patient underwent vascular surgery for repair of an abdominal aortic aneurysm.

Verbal: Spoken, using words.

Example: The paramedic called in a verbal report on the patient's condition to the emergency room nurse while transporting the patient to the hospital.

Virus: Microscopic infectious agent capable of replicating only in living cells, usually causing infectious disease.

Example: A person with a cold who goes shopping can transmit the virus to others.

Vital: Essential.

Example: The paramedic knows that it is vital to learn what type of poison was taken when caring for a poisoning victim.

Void: Excrete, or expel urine.

Example: The patient was instructed to void into the container so the nurse could observe the appearance of the urine.

Volume: Amount of space occupied by a fluid.

Example: The nurse recorded the volume of cough syrup administered to the patient.

REVIEW QUESTIONS

1. Select the meaning of the underlined word in the sentence. The client's condition was exacerbated in the fall.
   A. Improved
   B. Made worse
   C. Eliminated
   D. Created a scar

2. Select the meaning of the underlined word in the sentence. The overt signs of the baby's illness were distressing to the parents.
   A. Easily observed
   B. Subtle
   C. Intestinal
   D. Feverish

3. Select the meaning of the underlined word in the sentence. His paroxysmal coughing was a sign of this illness.
   A. Occasional
   B. Convulsive
   C. Discreet
   D. Soft

4. Select the meaning of the underlined word in the sentence. The bride decided to expand the number of people invited to the wedding.
   A. Decrease
   B. Increase
   C. Widen
   D. Reduce

5. Select the meaning of the underlined word in the sentence. The nurse noticed an abrupt change in the patient's level of pain.
   A. Slow
   B. Chronic
   C. Subtle
   D. Sudden

6. Select the meaning of the underlined word in the sentence. Her flushed appearance was noted by the nurse during the examination.
   A. Pale
   B. Excited
   C. Ruddy
   D. Indifferent

7. Select the meaning of the underlined word in the sentence. The nurse was keeping careful watch on the patient's respiration.
   A. Breathing
   B. Skin color
   C. Pulse
   D. Diet

8. Select the meaning of the underlined word in the sentence. The medication was given sublingually.
   A. By nasal inhaler
   B. By injection
   C. Under the tongue
   D. Under the eyelid

9. Select the meaning of the underlined word in the sentence. The rationale for the therapy was to increase the patient's range of motion.
   A. Prescription
   B. Outcome
   C. Goal
   D. Reason

10. Select the meaning of the underlined word in the sentence. The nurse is accountable for patient safety.
    A. Available
    B. Always aware
    C. Responsible
    D. Documenting

ANSWERS TO REVIEW QUESTIONS

1. B—Made worse
2. A—Easily observed
3. B—Convulsive
4. B—Increase
5. D—Sudden

6. C—Ruddy
7. A—Breathing
8. C—Under the tongue
9. D—Reason
10. C—Responsible

GRAMMAR

4

In the United States, the ability to speak and write the English language using proper grammar is a sign of an educated individual. When people are sick and need information or care from individuals in the health professions, they expect health care workers to be professional, well-educated individuals. It is therefore imperative that anyone in the health care professions understand and use proper grammar.

Grammar varies a great deal from language to language. English as a second language (ESL) students have an added burden to becoming successful. For example, nursing research literature indicates that ESL nursing students are at greater risk for attrition and failure of the licensing examination. However, this burden can be overcome by learning proper grammar.

CHAPTER OUTLINE

Eight Parts of Speech
Nine Important Terms to Understand
Ten Common Grammatical Mistakes

Four Suggestions for Success
Fifteen Troublesome Word Pairs
Summary

Review Questions
Answers to Review Questions

KEY TERMS

Adjective
Adverb
Clause (independent clause, dependent clause)
Cliché
Compound Sentence
Conjunction
Direct Object
Euphemism
Indirect Object

Interjection
Misplaced Modifier
Noun (common noun, proper noun, abstract noun, collective noun)
Participial Phrase
Participle
Phrase
Predicate
Predicate Adjective
Predicate Nominative

Preposition
Pronoun (personal pronoun, possessive pronoun)
Run-On Sentence
Sentence (declarative, interrogative, imperative, exclamatory)
Sentence Fragment
Sexist Language
Subject
Verb

This chapter describes the parts of speech, important terms and their uses in grammar, commonly occurring grammatical errors, and suggestions for successful use of grammar.

HESI Hint

From this day forward, listen only to English-speaking radio and television. If at all possible, speak only English at home and with friends.

Eight Parts of Speech

The eight parts of speech are nouns, pronouns, adjectives, verbs, adverbs, prepositions, conjunctions, and interjections.

Noun

A **noun** is a word or group of words that names a person, place, thing, or idea.

Common Noun A common noun is the general, not the particular, name of a person, place, or thing (e.g., *nurse, hospital, syringe*).

Proper Noun A proper noun is the official name of a person, place, or thing (e.g., *Fred, Paris, Washington University*). Proper nouns are capitalized.

Abstract Noun An abstract noun is the name of a quality or a general idea (e.g., *persistence, democracy*).

Collective Noun A collective noun is a noun that represents a group of persons, animals, or things (e.g., *family, flock, furniture*).

Pronoun

A **pronoun** is a word that takes the place of a noun, another pronoun, or a group of words acting as a noun. The word or group of words to which a pronoun refers is called the *antecedent*.

The *students* wanted *their* test papers graded and returned to *them* in a timely manner.

The word *students* is the antecedent of the pronouns *their* and *them*.

Personal Pronoun A personal pronoun refers to a specific person, place, thing, or idea by indicating the person speaking (first person), the person or people spoken to (second person), or any other person, place, thing, or idea being talked about (third person).

Personal pronouns also express number in that they are either singular or plural.

We [first person plural] were going to ask *you* [second person singular] to give *them* [third person plural] a ride to the office.

Possessive Pronoun A possessive pronoun is a form of personal pronoun that shows possession or ownership.

That is *my* book.
That book is *mine*.
That is *his* book.
That book is *his*.

A possessive pronoun does not contain an apostrophe.

HESI Hint

Do **not** use pronouns ending in *self* where they are inappropriate or unnecessary. *Use endings with self or selves only when there is a noun or personal pronoun in the sentence to refer back to.*
- I myself did the entire project.
- Sara did the entire project herself.

Notice that there are no such words as *hisself, theirself,* or *theirselves.*

Adjective

An **adjective** is a word, phrase, or clause that modifies a noun (the *biology* book) or pronoun (He is *nice*.). It answers the question *what kind* (a *hard* test), *which one* (an *English* test), *how many* (*three* tests), or *how much* (*many* tests). Verbs, pronouns, and nouns can act as adjectives. A type of verb form that functions as an adjective is a **participle**, which usually ends in -ing or -ed. Adjectives usually precede the noun or noun phrase that they modify (e.g., *the absent-minded professor*).

Examples

Verbs: The *scowling* professor, the *worried* student, the *broken* pencil

Pronouns: My book, *your* class, *that* book, *this* class

Nouns: The *professor's* class, the *biology* class

HESI Hint

Do **not** use the word *more* with certain adjectives, for example, those ending in *er*. It is improper grammar to say or to write *more better* or *more harder*. Likewise, do **not** use the word *most* with adjectives that end in *-est* or *-st*. It is improper grammar to say *most easiest* or *most worst*.

Verb

A **verb** is a word or phrase that is used to express an action or a state of being. A verb is the critical element of a sentence. Verbs express time through a property that is called the *tense*. The three primary tenses are:

- Present—Mary *works*
- Past—Mary *worked*
- Future—Mary *will work*

Some verbs are known as "linking verbs" because they link, or join, the subject of the sentence to a noun, pronoun, or predicate adjective. A linking verb does not show action.

- The most commonly used linking verbs are forms of the verb *to be: am, is, are, was, were, being, been* (e.g., That man *is* my professor.).
- Linking verbs are sometimes verbs that relate to the five senses: *look, sound, smell, feel,* and *taste* (e.g., That exam *looks* difficult.).
- Sometimes linking verbs reflect a state of being: *appear, seem, become, grow, turn, prove,* and *remain* (e.g., The professor *seems* tired.).

HESI Hint

The following are examples of proper and improper grammar related to verb usage:

It is important that Vanessa *send* **[not** *sends*] her resumé immediately.

I wish I were **[not** *was*] that smart.

If I were **[not** *was*] you, I'd leave now.

Adverb

An **adverb** is a word, phrase, or clause that modifies a verb, an adjective, or another adverb.

Examples

Verb: The physician operates *quickly*.

Adjective: The nurse wears *very* colorful uniforms.

Another Adverb: The student scored *quite* badly on the test.

Preposition

A **preposition** is a word that shows the relationship of a noun or pronoun to some other word in the sentence. A compound preposition is a preposition that is made up of more than one word. A prepositional phrase is a group of words that begins with a preposition and ends with a noun or a pronoun, which is called the *object* of the preposition. Box 4-1 lists commonly used prepositions.

Examples: Prepositional Phrases

Sam left the classroom *at noon*.

The students learned the basics *of grammar*.

Box 4-1   Commonly Used Prepositions

aboard	in
about	including
above	inside
across	into
after	like
against	minus
along	near
amid	of
among	off
around	on
as	onto
at	opposite
barring	out
before	outside
behind	over
below	past
beneath	pending
beside	plus
between	prior to
beyond	throughout
but (except)	to
by	toward
concerning	under
considering	underneath
despite	unlike
down	until
during	up
except	upon
following	with
for	within
from	without

Conjunction

A **conjunction** is a word that joins words, phrases, or clauses. Words that serve as *coordinating* conjunctions are *and, but, or, so, nor, for,* and *yet* (e.g., The nurse asked to work the early shift, *but* her request was denied.).

Correlative conjunctions work in pairs to join words or phrases (e.g., *Neither* the pharmacist *nor* her assistant could read the physician's handwriting.).

HESI Hint

Correlative conjunctions always stay in the same pairs. Two common pairs are *neither* and *nor* and *either* and *or*. These pairs should not be mixed; it is incorrect to use *neither* with *or* and *either* with *nor*. An easy way to remember this is to think that the two words that start with the letter "n" always go together.

Sometimes, subordinating conjunctions join two clauses or thoughts (e.g., *While* the nurse was away on vacation, the hospital flooded.). *While the nurse was away on vacation* is dependent on the rest of the sentence to complete its meaning.

Interjection

An **interjection** is a word or phrase that expresses emotion or exclamation. It does not have any grammatical connection to the other words in the sentence (e.g., *Yikes*, that test was hard. *Whew*, that test was easy.).

Nine Important Terms to Understand

There are nine important terms to understand: Clause, direct object, indirect object, phrase, predicate, predicate adjective, predicate nominative, sentence, and subject.

Clause

A **clause** is a group of words that has a subject and a predicate.

Independent Clause An independent clause expresses a complete thought and can stand alone as a sentence (e.g., *The professor distributed the examinations as soon as the students were seated.*). *The professor distributed the examinations* expresses a complete thought and can stand alone as a sentence.

Dependent Clause A dependent clause begins with a subordinating conjunction (Box 4-2) and does not express a complete thought and therefore cannot stand alone as a sentence. *As soon as the students were seated* does not express a complete thought. It needs the independent clause to complete the meaning and form the sentence.

HESI Hint

Independent clauses are used to write simple and compound sentences. Dependent clauses are added to an independent clause to form complex or compound-complex sentences. When a sentence begins with a dependent clause, use a comma to set it apart from the independent clause.

Box 4-2 Commonly Used Subordinating Conjunctions
after
because
before
until
since
when

Direct Object

A **direct object** is the person or thing that is directly affected by the action of the verb. A direct object answers the question *what* or *whom* after a transitive verb.

> The students watched the professor distribute the examinations.

> *The professor* answers *whom* the students watched.

Indirect Object

An **indirect object** is the person or thing that is indirectly affected by the action of the verb. A sentence can have an indirect object only if it has a direct object. An indirect object answers the question *to whom, for whom, to what,* or *for what* after an action verb.

> Indirect objects come between the verb and the direct object.

> The professor gave his class the test results.

> *His class* is the indirect object. It comes between the verb (*gave*) and the direct object (*test results*), and it answers the question *to whom.*

Phrase

A **phrase** is a group of two or more words that acts as a single part of speech in a sentence. A phrase can be used as a noun, an adjective, or an adverb. A phrase lacks a subject and a predicate.

Predicate

A **predicate** is the part of the sentence that tells what the subject does or what is done to the subject. It includes the verb and all the words that modify the verb.

Predicate Adjective

A **predicate adjective** follows a linking verb and helps to explain the subject.

> My professors are *wonderful.*

Predicate Nominative

A **predicate nominative** is a noun or pronoun that follows a linking verb and helps to explain or rename the subject.

> Professors are *teachers.*

Sentence

A **sentence** is a group of words that expresses a complete thought. Every sentence has a subject and a predicate. There are four types of sentences.

Declarative A declarative sentence makes a statement.

Example: I went to the store

Interrogative An interrogative sentence asks a question.

Example: Did you go to the store?

Imperative An imperative sentence makes a command or request.

Example: Go to the store.

Exclamatory An exclamatory sentence makes an exclamation.

Example: You went to the store!

HESI Hint

Many imperative sentences do not seem to have subjects. An imperative sentence usually has an implied subject. For example, when we say *Stop that now* the subject of the sentence, *you,* is implied *(You stop that now)*.

Subject

A **subject** is a word, phrase, or clause that names whom or what the sentence is about.

Ten Common Grammatical Mistakes

Subject-Verb Agreement

A subject must agree with its verb in number. A singular subject requires a singular verb. Likewise, a plural subject requires a plural verb.

Incorrect: The nurses (plural noun) *was* (singular verb) in a hurry to get there.

Correct: The nurses (plural noun) *were* (plural verb) in a hurry to get there.

There are times when the subject-verb agreement can be tricky to determine.

When the Subject and Verb Are Separated Find the subject and verb and make sure they agree.

Incorrect: The *question* that appears on all of the tests *are* inappropriate.

Correct: The *question* that appears on all of the tests *is* inappropriate.

Ignore any intervening phrases or clauses. Ignore words such as including, along with, as well as, together with, besides, except, and plus.

Example: The *dean*, along with his classes, *is* going on the tour of the facility.

Example: The *deans*, along with their classes, *are* going on the tour.

When the Subject Is a Collective Noun A collective noun is singular in form but plural in meaning. It is a noun that represents a group of persons, animals, or things (e.g., *family, audience, committee, board, faculty, herd, flock*).

If the group is acting as a single entity, use a singular verb.

Example: The *faculty agrees* to administer the test.

If the group is acting separately, use a plural verb.

Example: The *faculty are* not in agreement about which test to administer.

When the Subject Is a Compound Subject Usually, when the subject consists of two or more words that are connected by the word *and,* the subject is plural and calls for a plural verb.

Example: The *faculty* and the *students are* in the auditorium.

When the subject consists of two or more singular words that are connected by the words *or, either/or, neither/nor,* or *not only/but also,* the subject is singular and calls for a singular verb.

Example: Neither the *student* nor the *dean was* on time for class.

When the subject consists of singular and plural words that are connected by the words *or, either/or, neither/nor,* or *not only/but also,* choose a verb that agrees with the subject that is closest to the verb.

Example: Either the students or the teaching assistant is responsible.

Comma in a Compound Sentence

A **compound sentence** is a sentence that has two or more independent clauses. Each independent clause has a subject and a predicate and can stand alone as a sentence. When two independent clauses are joined by a coordinating conjunction such as *and, but, or,* or *nor,* place a comma before the conjunction.

Example: The professor thought the test was too easy, *but* the students thought it was too hard.

Run-On Sentence

A **run-on sentence** occurs when two or more complete sentences are written as though they were one sentence.

Example: The professor thought the test was too easy the students thought it was too hard.

A comma splice is one kind of run-on sentence. It occurs when two independent clauses are joined by only a comma.

Example: The professor thought the test was too easy, the students thought it was too hard.

The problem can be solved by replacing the comma with a dash, a semicolon, or a colon; by adding a coordinating conjunction; or by making two separate sentences.

Pronoun Case

Is it correct to say, "It was *me*" or "It was *I*"; "It must be *they*" or "It must be *them*"?

The correct pronoun to use depends on the pronoun's case. *Case* refers to the form of a noun or pronoun that indicates its relation to the other words in a sentence. There are three cases: *Nominative, objective,* and *possessive*. The case of a personal pronoun depends on the pronoun's function in the sentence. The pronoun can function as a subject, a complement (predicate nominative, direct object, or indirect object), an object of a preposition, or a replacement for a possessive noun.

Examples: Pronoun Use

- When the pronoun is the subject
  - *I* studied for the examination.
  - I is the subject of the sentence. Therefore use the nominative form of the pronoun.
- When pronouns are the subject in a compound subject
  - Is it correct to say, *"He and I went to the conference"* or *"Him and me went to the conference"*?
  - Is it accurate to say, *"John and me worked through the night"* or *"John and I worked through the night"*?
  - Is it proper to say, *"Her and Maria liked the chocolate-covered toffee"* or *"She and Maria liked the chocolate-covered toffee"*?

Knowing which pronoun is accurate requires understanding of how the pronoun is used in the sentence, so we know to use the nominative case. Therefore *He and I, I,* and *She* are the accurate forms of the pronouns.

HESI Hint

When choosing a pronoun that is in a compound subject, sometimes it is helpful to say the sentence without the conjunction and the other subject. We would not say, **Him** went to the conference or **Me** worked through the night or **Her** liked the chocolate-covered toffee. We would, however, say, **He** went to the conference and **I** worked through the night and **She** liked the chocolate-covered toffee.

HESI Hint

It is considered polite to place the pronoun *I* last in a series: *Luke, Jo, and **I** strive to do a good job.*

- When the pronoun is the object of the preposition

  Susan gave the results of the test to them.

  The pronoun *them* is the object of the preposition *to*. When the object of the preposition is a compound object as in *"Susan gave the results of the test to **Jo and me**,"* the objective form of the pronoun is used.
- When the pronoun replaces a possessive noun

  That desk is hers.

  The possessive pronoun *hers* is used to replace a possessive noun. For example, suppose there is a desk that belongs to Holly. We would say,

  That desk belongs to Holly. That is Holly's desk. That desk is Holly's. That desk is hers.

HESI Hint

Do not use an apostrophe with a possessive pronoun. There are no such words as *her's* or *their's.*

Pronouns that Indicate Possession

The possessive forms of personal pronouns have their own possessive forms, as shown in Table 4-1. Do not confuse these possessive pronouns with contractions that are similarly pronounced or spelled. Examples are shown in Table 4-2.

Table 4-1 Possessive Personal Pronouns

Pronoun	Possessive Forms	
I	My	Mine
He	His	His
She	Her	Hers
We	Our	Ours
You	Your	Yours
They	Their	Theirs
It	Its	Its

Table 4-2 Common Possessive Pronouns and Similar Contractions

Possessive Pronoun	Contraction
Its (belonging to *it*)	It's (it is, it has)
Their (belonging to *them*)	They're (they are)
Whose (belonging to *whom*)	Who's (who is, who has)
Your (belonging to *you*)	You're (you are)

Comma in a Series

Use a comma to separate three or more items in a series or list. A famous dedication makes the problem apparent: "To my parents, Ayn Rand and God." Because of the comma placement, it appears as though Ayn Rand and God are the parents. Place a comma between each item in the list and before the conjunction to avoid confusion.

Example: The nursing student took classes in English, biology, and chemistry.

Unclear or Vague Pronoun Reference

An unclear or vague pronoun reference makes a sentence confusing and difficult to understand.

Example: The teacher and the student knew that she was wrong.

Who was wrong: the teacher or the student? The meaning is unclear. Rewrite the sentence to avoid confusion.

Example: The teacher and the student knew that the *student* was wrong.

Sentence Fragments

Sentence fragments are incomplete sentences.

Example: While the students were taking the test.

The students were taking the test is a complete sentence. However, use of the word *while* turns it into a dependent clause. In order to make the fragment a sentence, it is necessary to supply an independent clause.

Example: While the students were taking the test, the professor walked around the classroom.

HESI Hint

Other words that commonly introduce dependent clauses are *among, because, although,* and *however.*

Misplaced Modifier

Misplaced modifiers are words or groups of words that are not located properly in relation to the words they modify.

Example: I fear my teaching assistant may have discarded the test I was grading in the trash can.

Was the test being graded in the trash can? The modifier *in the trash can* has been misplaced. The sentence should be rewritten so that the modifier is next to the word, phrase, or clause that it modifies.

Example: I fear the test I was grading may have been discarded in the trash can by my teaching assistant.

One type of misplaced modifier is a dangling participial phrase. A **participial phrase** is a phrase that is formed by a participle, its object, and the object's modifiers; the phrase functions as an adjective. A participial phrase modifies the noun that either directly precedes or directly follows the phrase. When the participial phrase directly precedes or directly follows a noun that it does not modify, the phrase is called a *dangling participial phrase.*

Example: Taking the patient's symptoms into account, a diagnosis was made by the physician.

The participial phrase *taking the patient's symptoms into account* is intended to modify the noun *physician;* however, because the phrase is placed closest to *diagnosis,* it appears to be modifying *diagnosis* instead of *physician.* Therefore the sentence as it is written states that the diagnosis took the patient's symptoms into account, which is impossible.

Example: Taking the patient's symptoms into account, the physician made a diagnosis.

Prepositions at the End of a Sentence

As a general rule, it is not very graceful to end a sentence with a preposition.

Example: Where in the world did that grammar rule come from?

Often an attempt to repair the error can result in a clumsy and awkward sentence.

Example: From where in the world did that grammar rule come?

Sometimes the sentence can be rewritten.

Example: Where in the world did that grammar rule originate?

Winston Churchill poked fun at the problem in response to those who objected to prepositions at the end of sentences: "This is the sort of English up with which I will not put."

Four Suggestions for Success

Eliminate Clichés

Clichés are expressions or ideas that have lost their originality or impact over time because of excessive use. Examples of clichés are *blind as a bat, dead as a doornail, flat as a pancake, raining cats and dogs, keep a stiff upper lip, let the cat out of the bag, sick as a dog, take the bull by the horns, under the weather, white as a sheet,* and *you can't judge a book by its cover.*

Clichés should be avoided whenever possible because they are old, tired, and overused. If tempted to use a cliché, endeavor to rephrase the idea.

Eliminate Euphemisms

A **euphemism** is a mild, indirect, or vague term that has been substituted for one that is considered harsh, blunt, or offensive. In many instances, euphemisms are used in a sympathetic manner to shield and protect. Some people refuse to refer to someone who has died as "dead." Instead, they say that the person has *passed away* or *gone to be with the Lord.* Euphemisms should be eliminated, and we should try to speak and write more accurately and honestly using our own words whenever appropriate.

It is also essential to use accurate and anatomically correct language when referring to the body, a body part, or a bodily function. To do otherwise is unprofessional and tactless.

Eliminate Sexist Language

Sexist language refers to spoken or written styles that do not satisfactorily reflect the presence of women in our society. Such language can suggest a sexist attitude on the part of the speaker or writer. Some believe that making men the default option is degrading and patronizing to women. In general, it is no longer considered appropriate to use *he* or *him* when referring to a hypothetical person. This can be especially important in contexts that refer to, for example, a physician as *he* or the nurse as *she.* In order to avoid such stereotypes, try to use gender-neutral titles that do not specify a particular gender. For example, use *firefighter* instead of *fireman, mail carrier* instead of *mailman, ancestors* instead of *forefathers, chair* instead of *chairman, supervisor* instead of *foreman,* *police officer* instead of *policeman,* and so on. Do not use terms such as *female doctor* or *male nurse* unless identifying the gender is necessary or appropriate. Similarly, do not use phrases such as *doctors and their wives;* use *doctors and their spouses* instead. If the idea is true that language shapes our thought processes, then we would do well to eliminate these sexist forms from our language.

HESI Hint

> Attempts to eliminate sexist language have created problems because often the word *his* is replaced with the word *their.* For example, *The doctor helps their patients.* However, this is grammatically incorrect because *their* is a plural pronoun that is being used in place of a singular noun. If the gender of the doctor is known, it is appropriate to use *his* or *her. The doctor helped her patients.* If the gender is not known, it is better to reword the sentence to avoid incorrect grammar, as well as sexist language.
> - Doctors help their patients.
> - The patients are helped by their doctor.

Eliminate Profanity and Insensitive Language

Insensitive and obscene language can be insulting and cruel. What we say does make a difference. The nursery rhyme we learned in our youth, "Sticks and stones may break my bones, but words will never hurt me," is simply not true. Ask anyone who has been on the receiving end of language that is patronizing or demeaning. Because language constantly changes, sometimes we can be offensive without even realizing that we have committed a blunder. In the age of an "anything goes" attitude for television, music lyrics, and the Internet, it is hard to know exactly what constitutes offensive language.

We need to be sensitive to language that excludes or emphasizes a person or group of people with reference to race, sexual orientation, age, gender, religion, or disability. We would all do well to remember another adage from childhood: The Golden Rule. Its message is clear: Respect the dignity of every human being, and treat others as you would like to be treated.

Fifteen Troublesome Word Pairs

Affect versus Effect

Affect is normally used as a verb that means "to influence or to change." (The chemotherapy *affected* [changed] my daily routine.) As a noun, *affect* is an emotional response or disposition. (The troubled teenager with the flat *affect* [disposition] attempted suicide.)

Effect may be used as a noun or a verb. As a noun, it means "result or outcome." (The chemotherapy had a strange *effect* [result] on me.) As a verb, it means "to bring about or accomplish." (As a result of the chemotherapy, I was able to *effect* [bring about] a number of changes in my life.)

Among versus Between

Use *among* to show a relationship involving more than two persons or things being considered as a group (The professor will distribute the textbooks *among* the students in his class).

Use *between* to show a relationship involving two persons or things (I sit *between* Holly and Jo in class), to compare one person or thing with an entire group (What's the difference between this book and other grammar books?), or to compare more than two things in a group if each is considered individually (I can't decide *between* the chemistry class, the biology class, and the anatomy class).

Amount versus Number

Amount is used when referring to things in bulk (The nurse had a huge *amount* of paperwork).

Number is used when referring to individual, countable units (The nurse had a *number* of charts to complete).

Good versus Well

Good is an adjective. Use *good* before nouns (He did a *good* job) and after linking verbs (She smells *good*) to modify the subject. *Well* is usually an adverb. When modifying a verb, use the adverb *well* (She plays softball *well*). *Well* is used as an adjective only when describing someone's health (She is getting *well*).

HESI Hint
To say that you feel well implies that you are in good health. To say that you are good or that you feel good implies that you are in good spirits.

Bad versus Badly

Apply the same rule for *bad* and *badly* that applies to good and well. Use *bad* as an adjective before nouns (He is a bad teacher) and after linking verbs (That smells bad) to modify the subject. Use *badly* as an adverb to modify an action verb (The student behaved *badly* in class).

HESI Hint
Do not use *badly* (or other adverbs) when using linking verbs that have to do with the senses. Say, "You felt *bad*." To say, "You felt *badly*" implies that something was wrong with your sense of touch. Say, "The mountain air smells wonderful." To say, "The mountain air smells wonderfully" implies that the air has a sense of smell that is used in a wonderful manner.

Bring versus Take

Bring conveys action toward the speaker—to carry from a distant place to a near place (Please *bring* your textbooks to class).

Take conveys action away from the speaker—to carry from a near place to a distant place (Please *take* your textbooks home).

Can versus May (Could versus Might)

Can and *could* imply ability or power (I *can* make an A in that class). *May* and *might* imply permission (You *may* leave early) or possibility (I *may* leave early).

Farther versus Further

Farther refers to a measurable distance (The walk to class is much *farther* than I expected). *Further* refers to a figurative distance and means "to a greater degree" or "to a greater extent" (I will have to study *further* to make better grades). *Further* also means "moreover" (Further/Furthermore, let me tell you something) and "in addition to" (The student had nothing *further* to say).

Fewer versus Less

Fewer refers to number—things that can be counted or numbered—and is used with plural nouns (The professor has *fewer* students in his morning class than he has in his afternoon class).

Less refers to degree or amount—things in bulk or in the abstract—and is used with singular nouns (*Fewer* patients mean *less* work for the staff). *Less* is also used when referring to numeric or statistical terms. (It's *less* than 2 miles to school. He scored *less* than 90 on the test. She spent *less* than $400 for this class. I am *less* than 5 feet tall.)

Hear versus Here

Hear is a verb meaning "to recognize sound by means of the ear" (Can you *hear* me now?). *Here* is most commonly used as an adverb meaning "at or in this place" (The test will be *here* tomorrow).

i.e. versus e.g.

The abbreviation *i.e.* (that is) is often confused with *e.g.* (for example); *i.e.* specifies or explains (I love to study chemistry, *i.e.*, the science dealing with the composition and properties of matter), and *e.g.* gives an example. (I love to study chemistry, *e.g.*, chemical equations, atomic structure, and molar relationships.)

Learn versus Teach

Learn means "to receive or acquire knowledge" (I am going to *learn* all that I can about nursing). *Teach* means "to give or impart knowledge" (I will *teach* you how to convert decimals to fractions).

Lie versus Lay

Lie means "to recline or rest." The principal parts of the verb are *lie, lay, lain,* and *lying*. Forms of *lie* are never followed by a direct object.

Examples

- I *lie* down to rest.
- I *lay* down yesterday to rest.
- I had *lain* down to rest.
- I was *lying* on the sofa.

Lay means "to put or place." The principal parts of the verb are *lay, laid, laid,* and *laying*. Forms of *lay* are followed by a direct object.

Examples

- I *lay* the book on the table.
- I *laid* the book on the table yesterday.
- I have *laid* the book on the table before.
- I am *laying* the book on the table now.

HESI Hint

To help determine whether the use of *lie* or *lay* is appropriate in a sentence, substitute the word in question with "place, placed, placing" (whichever is appropriate). If the substituted word makes sense, the equivalent form of *lay* is correct. If the sentence doesn't make sense with the substitution, the equivalent form of *lie* is correct.

Which versus That

Which is used to introduce nonessential clauses, and *that* is used to introduce essential clauses. A nonessential clause adds information to the sentence but is not necessary to make the meaning of the sentence clear. Use commas to set off a nonessential clause. An essential clause adds information to the sentence that is needed to make the sentence clear. Do not use commas to set off an essential clause

Example: The hospital, *which flooded last July*, is down the street.

In this case, the phrase *which flooded last July* is a nonessential clause that is simply providing more information about the hospital.

Example: The hospital *that flooded last July* is down the street; the other hospital is across town.

In this case, the phrase *that flooded last July* is an essential clause because the information distinguishes the two hospitals as the one that flooded and the one that did not.

Who versus Whom

Who and *whom* serve as interrogative pronouns and relative pronouns. An interrogative pronoun is one that is used to form questions, and a relative pronoun is one that relates groups of words to nouns or other pronouns.

Examples

- *Who* is getting an A in this class? (Interrogative)
- Susan is the one *who* is getting an A in this class. (Relative)
- To *whom* shall I give the textbook? (Interrogative)
- Susan, *whom* the professor favors, is very bright. (Relative)

Who and *whom* may be singular or plural.

Examples

- *Who* is getting an A in this class? (Singular)
- *Who* are the students getting As in this class? (Plural)
- *Whom* did you say is passing the class? (Singular)
- *Whom* did you say are passing the class? (Plural)

Who is the nominative case. Use it for subjects and predicate nominatives.

HESI Hint

Use *who* or *whoever* if *he, she, they, I,* or *we* can be substituted in the *who* clause.

Who passed the chemistry test? *He/she/they/I* passed the chemistry test.

Whom is the objective case. Use it for direct objects, indirect objects, and objects of the prepositions.

HESI Hint

Use *whom* or *whomever* if *him, her, them, me,* or *us* can be substituted as the object of the verb or as the object of the preposition in the *whom* clause.

To *whom* did the professor give the test? He gave the test to *him/her/them/me/us.*

Summary

Review this chapter and ask yourself whether your use of the English language reflects that of an educated individual. If so, congratulations! If not, study the content of this chapter, and your scores on the HESI Admission Assessment are likely to improve.

REVIEW QUESTIONS

1. Which of the following sentences is grammatically incorrect?
   A. We took him to the store, the library, and the restaurant.
   B. We took him to the store and the library.
   C. We took him to the store and then we went to the library.
   D. We took him to the store and then went to the library.

2. Select the best word for the blank in the following sentence.
   I will _____ that chart to the patient's room later today.
   A. Bring
   B. Take
   C. Brought
   D. Took

3. Which word in the following sentence should be replaced?
   The department chairman stepped up to the podium.
   A. Podium
   B. Stepped
   C. Chairman
   D. Up

4. Which word in the following sentence is an indirect object?
   The doctor gave the patient a prescription.
   A. Doctor
   B. Prescription
   C. Gave
   D. Patient

5. Which of the following sentences is grammatically correct?
   A. The patient and the nurse knew that he could walk.
   B. While the patient was walking.
   C. The patient, the nurse and the doctor were walking.
   D. Because the patient could walk, he was allowed to leave his room.

6. Which of the following sentences is grammatically correct?
   A. The child's torn shirt was laying on the floor.
   B. The torn child's shirt was laying on the floor.
   C. The child's shirt was laying on the floor torn.
   D. The child's shirt torn was laying on the floor.

7. Which of the following sentences contains an interjection?
   A. I hope you have finished digging your well.
   B. I hope you are feeling well.
   C. Well, I hope you are happy.
   D. I hope you perform well on the test.

8. Which word is used incorrectly in the following sentence?
   To who should the letter be addressed?
   A. Who
   B. Should
   C. Letter
   D. Addressed

9. Select the best word for the blank in the following sentence.

   He couldn't _____ the speaker's words because of the nearby airport noise.
   A. here
   B. hear
   C. comprehend
   D. understand

10. What word is used incorrectly in this sentence?

    The six students in the class discussed the test results between themselves.
    A. discussed
    B. results
    C. between
    D. themselves

ANSWERS TO REVIEW QUESTIONS

1. C—"We took him to the store" and "then we went to the library" are two independent clauses joined by the conjunction "and." Therefore there should be a comma after the word "store." The correct sentence is "We took him to the store, and then we went to the library."
2. B—In this sentence, the action is away from the speaker, who will carry the patient's chart from a near place (where the speaker is) to a far place (the patient's room). Therefore the best word is "take."
3. C—The word "chairman" is considered sexist language. Sexist language can be avoided by changing *chairman* to *chair* or *chairperson*.
4. D—The indirect object is the person or thing indirectly affected by the action of the verb. In this sentence, patient is the indirect object. Indirect objects come between the verb and the direct object.
5. D—D is the only sentence that is grammatically correct. A includes a vague pronoun reference (does *he* refer to the patient or to the nurse?). B is a sentence fragment. C includes a series, and there should be a comma after *nurse*.
6. A—*Torn* is modifying *shirt*, so it should be placed next to shirt. In B, C, and D, the modifier is misplaced.
7. C—In this sentence *well* expresses emotion and does not have a grammatical connection to the rest of the sentence.
8. A—*Who* should be *whom* in this sentence because it is the object of the preposition *to*.
9. B—*Hear* means to recognize sound by means of the ear. *Here* is a site differentiation. C and D would fit in the sentence, but the reference to airport noise makes B the best choice.
10. C—*Between* implies only two people. The correct word to use in the sentence would be *among*. A, B, and D are used correctly.

BIOLOGY

5

Biology is the scientific study of life. Members of the health professions naturally deal with biology, whether it requires knowing the structure of a cell, understanding how a molecule will react to a medication or treatment, or comprehending how certain organisms in the body function. Prospective students desiring to enter one of the health professions should have a basic knowledge of biology.

This chapter reviews the structure and reactions of cells and molecules. The concepts of cellular respiration, photosynthesis, cellular reproduction, and genetics are also presented.

CHAPTER OUTLINE

Biology Basics
Water
Biologic Molecules
Metabolism

The Cell
Cellular Respiration
Photosynthesis
Cellular Reproduction

Genetics
DNA
Review Questions
Answers to Review Questions

KEY TERMS

Alleles
Amino Acids
Binary Fission
Chromosomes
Codon
Cytokinesis
Deoxyribonucleic Acid (DNA)
Electron Transport Chain
Glycolysis
Golgi Apparatus
Heterozygous

Homozygous
Interphase
Krebs Cycle
Meiosis
Messenger RNA (mRNA)
Metabolic Pathway
Metaphase Plate
Mitosis
Organelles
Phagocytosis
Phospholipids

Photosynthesis
Punnett Square
Ribonucleic Acid (RNA)
Rough ER
Smooth ER
Steroids
Stop Codon
Transcription
Transfer RNA (tRNA)

Biology Basics

In biology, there is a hierarchic system of organization. The system is most inclusive as kingdom and least as species. The order is as follows:

- Kingdom
- Phylum
- Class
- Order
- Family
- Genus
- Species

Most scientists agree that the core theme in biology today is the idea of evolution. Charles Darwin first introduced this notion in 1859 in his book *On the Origin of Species.* He proposed that current species arose from a process he called "descent with modification."

Science is a process. For an experiment to be performed, the following steps must be taken:

- The first step is hypothesis, which is a statement or explanation of certain events or happenings.
- The second step is the experiment, which is a repeatable procedure of gathering data to support or refute the hypothesis.
- The final step in the scientific process is the conclusion.

Water

Water is the substance that makes life possible. The molecule itself is simply two hydrogen atoms covalently bonded to one oxygen atom. The most significant aspect of water is the polarity of its bonds.

It is the polar nature of water that allows for hydrogen bonding between molecules. This type of intermolecular bonding has several resulting benefits. The first of these is water's high specific heat.

The specific heat of a molecule is the amount of heat necessary to raise the temperature of 1 gram of that molecule by 1° Celsius. Water has a relatively high specific heat value, which allows water to resist shifts in temperature. One powerful benefit is the ability of oceans or large bodies of water to stabilize climates.

Hydrogen bonding also results in strong cohesive and adhesive properties. Cohesion is the ability of a molecule to stay bonded or attracted to another molecule of the same substance. A good example is how water tends to run together on a newly waxed car. Adhesion is the ability of water to bond to or attract other molecules or substances. When water is sprayed on a wall, some of it sticks to the wall. That is adhesion.

When water freezes, it forms a lattice, which actually causes the molecules to spread apart, resulting in the phenomenon of floating. Most molecules, when they are in the solid form, do not float on the liquid form of the substance. If ice did not float, lakes would freeze from the bottom to the top. Life could not exist as we know it.

The polarity of water also allows it to act as a versatile solvent. Water can be used to dissolve a number of different substances (Figure 5-1).

Biologic Molecules

There are multitudes of molecules that are significant to biology. The most important molecules are carbohydrates, lipids, proteins, and nucleic acids.

Carbohydrates

Carbohydrates are generally long chains, or polymers, of sugars. They have many functions and serve many different purposes. The most important of these are storage, structure, and energy.

Lipids

Lipids are better known as fats, but specifically they are fatty acids, phospholipids, and steroids.

Fatty Acids Fatty acids vary greatly but simply are grouped into two categories: saturated and unsaturated. Saturated fats contain no double bonds in their hydrocarbon tail. Conversely, unsaturated fats have one or more double bonds. As a result, saturated fats are solid, whereas unsaturated fats are liquid at room temperature. Saturated fats are those the general public considers detrimental; cardiovascular problems are likely with diets that contain high quantities of saturated fats.

Phospholipids Phospholipids consist of two fatty acids of varying length bonded to a phosphate group. The phosphate group is charged and therefore polar, whereas the hydrocarbon tail of the fatty acids is nonpolar. This quality is particularly important in the function of cellular membranes. The molecules combine in a way that creates a barrier that protects the cell.

Steroids The last of the lipids are **steroids.** They are a component of membranes, but more important, many are precursors to significant hormones.

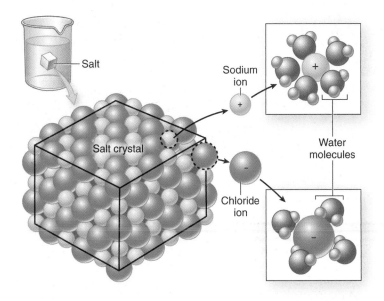

FIGURE 5-1 Water as a solvent. The polar nature of water *(blue)* favors ionization of substances in solution. Sodium (Na$^+$) ions *(pink)* and chloride (Cl$^-$) ions *(green)* dissociate in the solution. (From Patton KT, Thibodeau GA: *Anatomy and physiology,* ed 7, St Louis, 2010, Mosby.)

Proteins

Proteins are the most significant contributor to cellular function. They are polymers of 20 molecules called **amino acids.** Proteins are complex, consist of several structure types, and are the largest of the biologic molecules. Enzymes are particular types of proteins that act to catalyze different reactions or processes. Nearly all cellular function is catalyzed by some type of enzyme.

Nucleic Acids

Nucleic acids are components of the molecules of inheritance. **Deoxyribonucleic acid (DNA)** is a unique molecule specific to a particular organism and contains the code that is necessary for replication (Figure 5-2). **Ribonucleic acid (RNA)** is used in transfer and as a messenger in most species of the genetic code.

Metabolism

Metabolism is the sum of all chemical reactions that occur in an organism. In a cell, reactions take place in a series of steps called **metabolic pathways,** progressing from a standpoint of high energy to low energy. All of the reactions are catalyzed by the use of enzymes.

The Cell

The cell is the fundamental unit of biology. There are two types of cells: prokaryotic and eukaryotic cells. Cells consist of many components, most of which are referred to as **organelles.** Figure 5-3 illustrates a typical cell.

Prokaryotic cells lack a defined nucleus and do not contain membrane-bound organelles. Eukaryotic cells have a membrane-enclosed nucleus and a series of membrane-bound organelles that carry out the functions of the cell as directed by the nucleus. In other words, prokaryotic cells do not have membrane-bound organelles, whereas eukaryotic cells do. The eukaryotic cell is the more complex of the two cell types.

There are several different organelles functioning in a cell at a given time; only the major ones are considered here.

Nucleus

The first of the organelles is the nucleus, which contains the DNA of the cell in organized masses called **chromosomes.** Chromosomes contain all of the material for the regeneration of the cell, as well as all instructions for the function of the cell. Every organism has a characteristic number of chromosomes specific to the particular species.

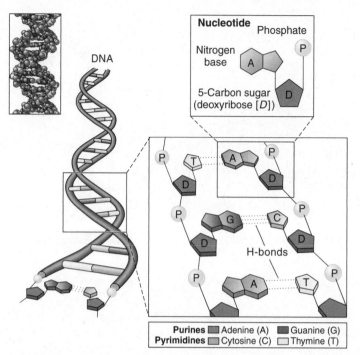

FIGURE 5-2   The DNA molecule. Representation of the DNA double helix showing the general structure of a nucleotide and the two kinds of "base pairs": adenine (A) *(blue)* with thymine (T) *(yellow)* and guanine (G) *(purple)* with cytosine (C) *(red)*. Note that the G–C base pair has three hydrogen bonds and an A–T base pair has two. Hydrogen bonds are extremely important in maintaining the structure of this molecule. (From Patton KT, Thibodeau GA: *Anatomy and physiology*, ed 7, St Louis, 2010, Mosby.)

Ribosomes

Ribosomes are organelles that read the RNA produced in the nucleus and translate the genetic instructions to produce proteins. Cells with a high rate of protein synthesis generally have a large number of ribosomes. Ribosomes can be found in two locations. Bound ribosomes are those found attached to the endoplasmic reticulum (ER), and free ribosomes are those found in the cytoplasm. The two types are interchangeable and have identical structures, although they have slightly different roles.

Endoplasmic Reticulum

The ER is a membranous organelle found attached to the nuclear membrane and consists of two continuous parts. Through an electron microscope, it is clear that part of the membranous system is covered with ribosomes. This section of the ER is referred to as **rough ER,** and it is responsible for protein synthesis and membrane production. The other section of the ER lacks ribosomes and is referred to as **smooth ER.** It

functions as the detoxification and metabolism of multiple molecules.

Golgi Apparatus

Inside the cell is a packaging, processing, and shipping organelle that is called the **Golgi apparatus.** The Golgi apparatus transports materials from the ER throughout the cell.

Lysosomes

Intracellular digestion takes place in lysosomes. Packed with hydrolytic enzymes, the lysosomes can hydrolyze proteins, fats, sugars, and nucleic acids.

Vacuoles

Vacuoles are membrane-enclosed structures that have various functions, depending on cell type. Many cells, through a process called **phagocytosis,** uptake food through the cell membrane, creating a

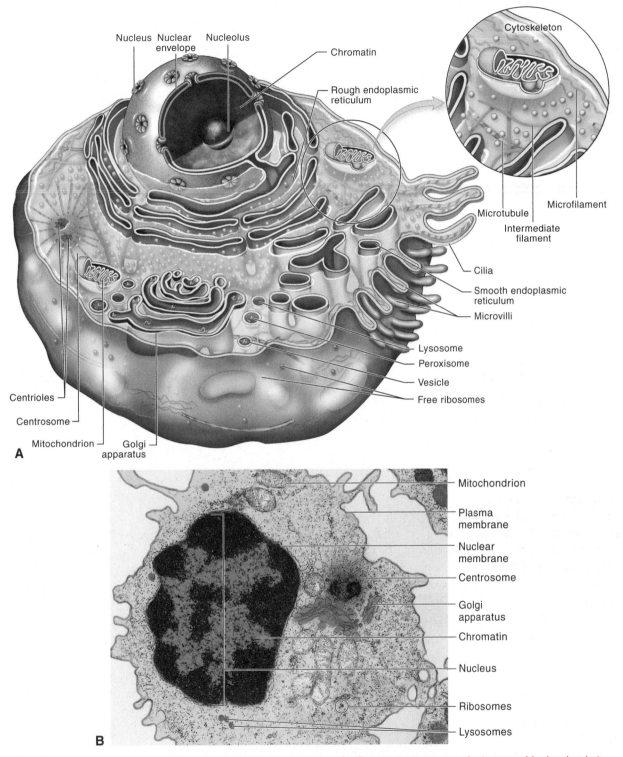

FIGURE 5-3   Typical, or composite, cell. **A,** Artist's interpretation of cell structure. Note, too, the innumerable dots bordering the endoplasmic reticulum. These are ribosomes, the cell's "protein factories." **B,** Color-enhanced electron micrograph of a cell. Both show the many mitochondria, known as the "power plants of the cell." Note, too, the innumerable dots bordering the endoplasmic reticulum. These are ribosomes, the cell's "protein factories." (From Patton KT, Thibodeau GA: *Anatomy and physiology,* ed 7, St Louis, 2010, Mosby. **B,** Courtesy A. Arlan Hinchee.)

food vacuole. Plant cells have a central vacuole that functions as storage, waste disposal, protection, and hydrolysis.

Mitochondria and Chloroplasts

There are two distinct organelles that produce cell energy: the mitochondrion and the chloroplast. Mitochondria are found in most eukaryotic cells and are the site of cellular respiration. Chloroplasts are found in plants and are the site of photosynthesis.

Cellular Membrane

The cellular membrane is the most important component of the cell, contributing to protection, communication, and the passage of substances into and out of the cell. The cell membrane itself consists of a bilayer of phospholipids with proteins, cholesterol, and glycoproteins peppered throughout. Because phospholipids are amphipathic molecules, this bilayer creates a hydrophobic region between the two layers of lipids, making it selectively permeable. Many of the proteins, which pass completely through the membrane, act as transport highways for molecular movement into and out of the cell. Figure 5-4 illustrates the structure of the cellular membrane.

Cellular Respiration

There are two catabolic pathways that lead to cellular energy production. As a simple combustion reaction, cellular respiration produces far

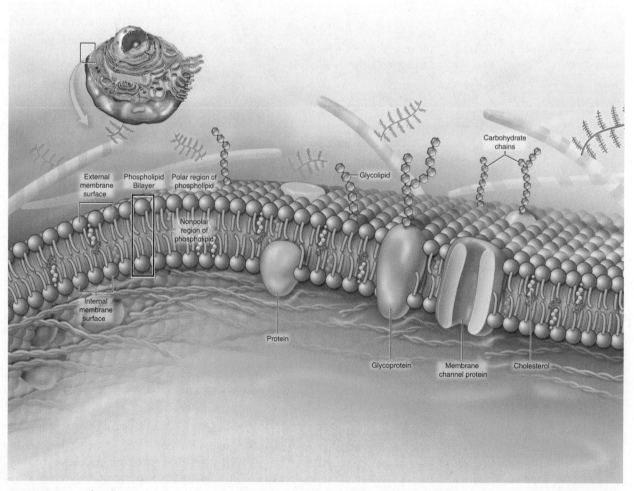

FIGURE 5-4 The plasma membrane is made of a bilayer of phospholipid molecules arranged with their nonpolar "tails" pointing toward each other. Cholesterol molecules help stabilize the flexible bilayer structure to prevent breakage. Protein molecules and protein-hybrid molecules may be found on the outer or inner surface of the bilayer—or extending all the way through the membrane. (From Patton KT, Thibodeau GA: *Anatomy and physiology*, ed 7, St Louis, 2010, Mosby.)

more energy than does its anaerobic counterpart, fermentation.

$$C_6H_{12}O_6 + 6O_2 \rightarrow 6CO_2 + 6H_2O$$

This balanced equation is the simplified chemistry behind respiration. The process itself actually occurs in a series of three complex steps that are simplified for our purposes.

There is one molecule that is used as the currency of the cell: adenosine triphosphate (ATP). Another compound that acts as a reducing agent and is a vehicle of stored energy is reduced nicotinamide adenine dinucleotide (NADH). This molecule is used as a precursor to produce greater amounts of ATP in the final steps of respiration.

The first step is the conversion of glucose to pyruvate in a process called **glycolysis.** It takes place in the cytosol of the cell and produces two molecules of ATP, two molecules of pyruvate, and two molecules of NADH.

In step two, the pyruvate is transported into a mitochondrion and used in the first of a series of reactions called the **Krebs cycle.** This cycle takes place in the matrix of the mitochondria, and for a single consumed glucose molecule, two ATP molecules, six molecules of carbon dioxide, and six NADH molecules are produced.

The third step begins with the oxidation of the NADH molecules to produce oxygen and finally to produce water in a series of steps called the **electron transport chain.** The energy harvest here is remarkable. For every glucose molecule, 28 to 32 ATP molecules can be produced.

This conversion results in overall ATP production numbers of 32 to 36 ATP molecules for every glucose molecule consumed. For a summary of cellular respiration, see Figure 5-5.

Photosynthesis

In the previous section the harvesting of energy by the cell was discussed. But where did that energy originate? It began with a glucose molecule and resulted in a large production of energy in the form of ATP. A precursor to the glucose molecule is produced in a process called **photosynthesis.**

The chemical reaction representing this process is simply the reverse of cellular respiration.

$$6CO_2 + 6H_2O + \text{Light energy} \rightarrow C_6H_{12}O_6 + 6O_2$$

The only notable difference is the addition of light energy on the reactant side of the equation.

Just as glucose is used to produce energy, so too must energy be used to produce glucose.

Photosynthesis is not as simple a process as it looks from the chemical equation. In fact, it consists of two different stages: the light reactions and the Calvin cycle. The light reactions are those that convert solar energy to chemical energy. The cell accomplishes the production of ATP by absorbing light and using that energy to split a water molecule and transfer the electron, thus creating nicotinamide adenine dinucleotide phosphate (NADPH) and producing ATP. These molecules are then used in the Calvin cycle to produce sugar.

The sugar produced is polymerized and stored as a polymer of glucose. These sugars are consumed by organisms or by the plant itself to produce energy by cellular respiration.

HESI Hint

When attempting to understand cell respiration and photosynthesis, keep in mind that these processes are cyclical. In other words, the raw materials for one process are the products of the other process. The raw materials for cell respiration are glucose and oxygen, whereas the products of cell respiration are water, carbon dioxide, and ATP. Plants and other autotrophs will utilize the products of cell respiration in the process of photosynthesis. The products of photosynthesis (oxygen, glucose) become the raw materials of cell respiration.

Cellular Reproduction

Cells reproduce by three different processes, all of which fall into two categories: sexual and asexual reproduction.

Asexual Reproduction

There are two types of asexual reproduction. The first involves bacterial cells and is referred to as **binary fission.** In this process, the chromosome binds to the plasma membrane, where it replicates. Then as the cell grows, it pinches in two, producing two identical cells (Figure 5-6).

Another type of asexual reproduction is called **mitosis.** This process of cell division occurs in five stages before pinching in two in a process called **cytokinesis.** The five stages are prophase, prometaphase, metaphase, anaphase, and telophase.

During prophase, the chromosomes are visibly separate, and each duplicated chromosome has

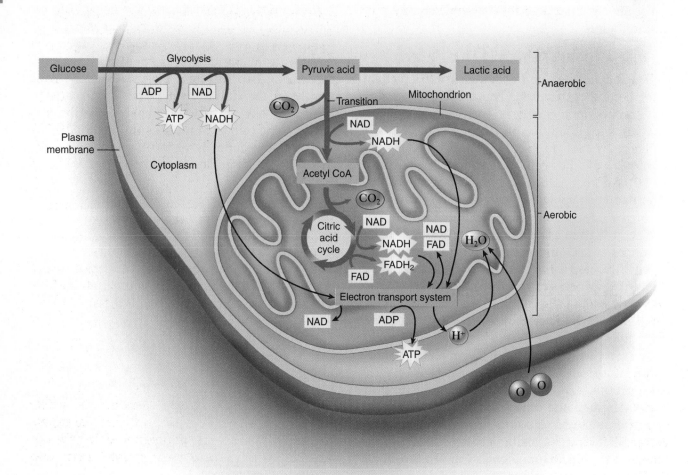

FIGURE 5-5 Summary of cellular respiration. This simplified outline of cellular respiration represents one of the most important catabolic pathways in the cell. Note that one phase *(glycolysis)* occurs in the cytosol but that the two remaining phases (*citric acid cycle* and *electron transport system*) occur within a mitochondrion. Note also the divergence of the anaerobic and aerobic pathways of cellular respiration. *ADP*, Adenosine diphosphate; *ATP*, adenosine triphosphate; *CoA*, coenzyme A; *FAD*, flavin adenine dinucleotide; *FADH₂,* form of flavin adenine dinucleotide; *NAD*, nicotinamide adenine dinucleotide; *NADH*, form of nicotinamide adenine dinucleotide. (From Patton KT, Thibodeau GA: *Anatomy and physiology,* ed 7, St Louis, 2010, Mosby.)

two noticeable sister chromatids. In prometaphase, the nuclear envelope begins to disappear, and the chromosomes begin to attach to the spindle that is forming along the axis of the cell. Metaphase follows, with all the chromosomes aligning along what is called the **metaphase plate,** or the center of the cell. Anaphase begins when chromosomes start to separate. In this phase, the chromatids are considered separate chromosomes. The final phase is telophase. Here, chromosomes gather on either side of the now separating cell. This is the end of mitosis.

The second process associated with cell division is cytokinesis. During this phase, which is separate from the phases of mitosis, the cell pinches in two, forming two separate identical cells. A summary of mitosis is illustrated in Figure 5-7.

Sexual Reproduction

Sexual reproduction is different from asexual reproduction. In asexual reproduction, the offspring originates from a single cell, yielding all

Binary fission in bacteria

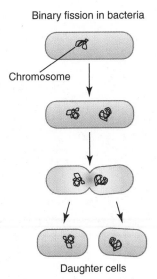

Chromosome

Daughter cells

FIGURE 5-6 Binary fission. A single cell separates into two identical daughter cells, each with an identical copy of parent DNA. (Redrawn from VanMeter K, et al: *Microbiology for the healthcare professional,* St. Louis, 2010, Mosby.)

cells produced to be identical. In sexual reproduction, two cells contribute genetic material to the daughter cells, resulting in significantly greater variation. These two cells find and fertilize each other randomly, making it virtually impossible for cells to be alike.

The process that determines how reproductive cells divide in a sexually reproducing organism is called **meiosis.** Meiosis consists of two distinct stages, meiosis one and meiosis two, resulting in four daughter cells (Figure 5-8). Each of these daughter cells contains half as many chromosomes as the parent. Preceding these events is a period called **interphase.** It is during interphase that the chromosomes are duplicated and the cell prepares for division.

HESI Hint

Meiosis versus Mitosis

To illustrate the need for a reduction division (meiosis) in sex cell production, calculate the chromosome numbers that would result if sperm and egg cells were produced by mitosis. If both sperm and eggs were the result of mitosis, their chromosome number would be 46 not 23. At fertilization, the chromosome number of the zygote would be 92, and the gametes produced by such an individual would also have 92 chromosomes. Of course, a zygote resulting from the fertilization of

gametes containing 92 chromosomes would have a chromosome number of 184. The need to produce gametes by meiotic and not mitotic division soon becomes obvious.

The first stage of meiosis consists of four phases: prophase I, metaphase I, anaphase I, and telophase I and cytokinesis. The significant differences between meiosis and mitosis occur in prophase I. During this phase, nonsister chromatids of homologous chromosomes cross at numerous locations. Small sections of DNA are transferred between these chromosomes, resulting in increased genetic variation. The remaining three phases are the same as those in mitosis, with the exception that the chromosome pairs separate, not the chromosomes themselves.

After the first cytokinesis, meiosis two begins. Here, all four stages, identical to those of mitosis, occur. The resulting four cells have half as many chromosomes as the parent cell.

Genetics

Using garden peas, Gregor Mendel discovered the basic principles of genetics. By careful experimentation, he was able to determine that the observable traits in peas were passed from one generation to the next.

From Mendel's studies, scientists have found that for every trait expressed in a sexually reproducing organism, there are at least two alternative versions of a gene, called **alleles.** For simple traits, the versions can be one of two types: dominant or recessive. If both of the alleles are the same type, the organism is said to be **homozygous** for that trait. If they are different types, the organism is said to be **heterozygous.**

HESI Hint

If an allele is dominant for a particular trait, the letter chosen to represent that allele is capitalized. If the allele is recessive, then the letter is lowercased. If a dominant allele is present, then the phenotype expressed will be the dominant. The only way a recessive trait will be expressed is if both alleles are recessive.

By use of a device called a **Punnett square,** it is possible to predict genotype (the combination of alleles) and phenotype (what traits will be expressed) of the offspring of sexual reproduction.

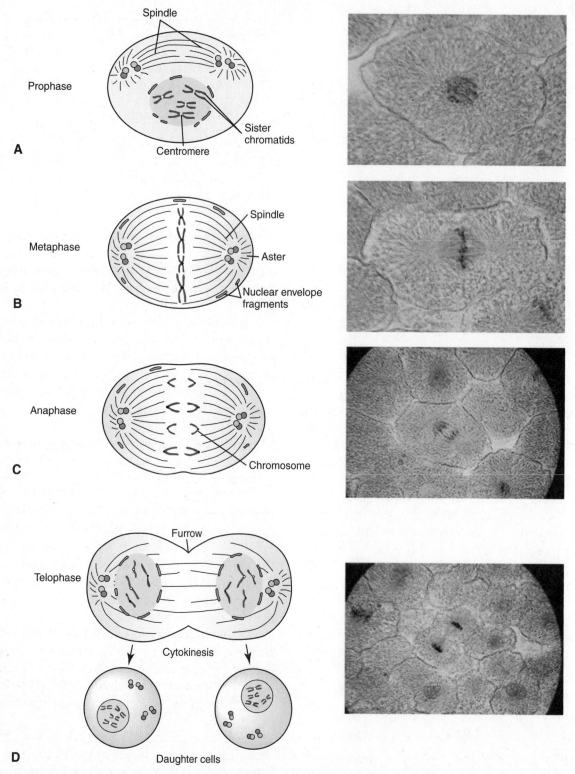

FIGURE 5-7 Mitosis. **A,** Prophase. **B,** Metaphase. **C,** Anaphase. **D,** Telophase. (Redrawn from VanMeter K, et al: *Microbiology for the healthcare professional*, St. Louis, 2010, Mosby.)

	R	r
R	RR	Rr
r	Rr	rr

FIGURE 5-10   Punnett square depicting three possible dominant combinations.

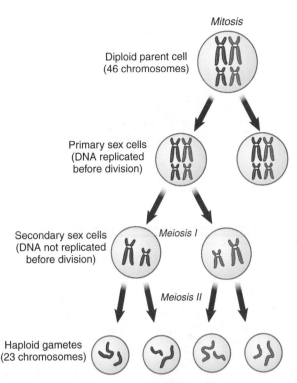

Mitosis

Diploid parent cell
(46 chromosomes)

Primary sex cells
(DNA replicated
before division)

Meiosis I

Secondary sex cells
(DNA not replicated
before division)

Meiosis II

Haploid gametes
(23 chromosomes)

FIGURE 5-8   Meiosis. Meiotic cell division takes place in two steps: *meiosis I* and *meiosis II.* Meiosis is called *reduction division* because the number of chromosomes is reduced by half (from the diploid number to the haploid number). (From Patton KT, Thibodeau GA: *Anatomy and physiology,* ed 7, St Louis, 2010, Mosby.)

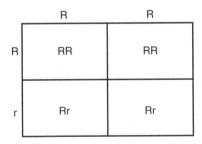

	R	R
R	RR	RR
r	Rr	Rr

FIGURE 5-9   Punnett square depicting the cross between a homozygous dominant and a heterozygous organism.

Alleles are placed one per column for one gene and one per row for the other gene. In the example in Figure 5-9, a homozygous dominant is crossed with a heterozygous organism for the same trait. Note that all progeny will express dominance for this trait. In the example in Figure 5-10, three of the possible combinations will be dominant, and one will be recessive for this trait.

The Punnett square can be used to cross any number of different traits simultaneously. With these data, a probability of phenotypes that will be produced can be determined. However, the more traits desired, the more complex the cross.

Not all genes express themselves according to these simple rules, but they are the basis for all genetic understanding. There are many other methods of genetic expression. A few of these include multiple alleles, pleiotropy, epistasis, and polygenic inheritance.

Because genetics is the study of heredity, many human disorders can be detected by studying a person's chromosomes or by creating a pedigree. A pedigree is a family tree that traces the occurrence of a certain trait through several generations. A pedigree is useful in understanding the genetic past as well as the possible future.

DNA

DNA is the genetic material of a cell and is the vehicle of inheritance. In 1953, Watson and Crick described the structure of DNA. They described a double helical structure that contains the four nitrogenous bases adenine, thymine, guanine, and cytosine.

Each base forms hydrogen bonds with another base on the complementary strand. The bases have a specific bonding pattern. Adenine bonds with thymine, and guanine bonds with cytosine. Because of this method of bonding, the strands can be replicated, producing identical strands of DNA. During replication, the strands are separated. Then, with the help of several enzymes, new complementary strands to each of the two original strands are created. This produces two new double-stranded segments of DNA identical to the original (Figure 5-11).

Each gene along a strand of DNA is a template for protein synthesis. This production begins with a process called **transcription.** In this process, an RNA strand, complementary to the original strand of DNA, is produced. The piece of genetic material produced is called **messenger RNA (mRNA).** The RNA strand has nitrogenous bases identical to those in DNA with the exception of uracil, which is substituted for thymine.

mRNA functions as a messenger from the original DNA helix in the nucleus to the ribosomes in the cytosol or on the rough ER. Here, the ribosome acts as the site of translation. The mRNA slides through the ribosome. Every group of three bases along the stretch of RNA is called a **codon,** and each of these codes for a specific amino acid. The anticodon is located on a unit called **transfer RNA (tRNA),** which carries a specific amino acid. It binds to the ribosome when its codon is sliding through the ribosome. Remember that a protein is a polymer of amino acids, and multiple tRNA molecules bind in order and are released by the ribosome. Each amino acid is bonded together and released by the preceding tRNA molecule, creating an elongated chain of amino acids. Eventually the chain is ended at what is called a **stop codon.** At this point, the chain is released into the cytoplasm, and the protein folds onto itself and forms its complete conformation.

By dictating what is produced in translation through transcription, the DNA in the nucleus has control over everything taking place in the cell. The proteins that are produced will perform all the different cellular functions required for the cell's survival. The synthesis of proteins is summarized in Figure 5-12.

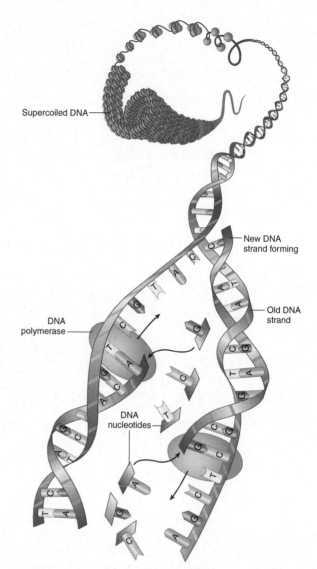

FIGURE 5-11 DNA replication. When a DNA molecule makes a copy of itself, it "unzips" to expose its nucleotide bases. Through the mechanism of obligatory base pairing, coordinated by the enzyme *DNA polymerase,* new DNA nucleotides bind to the exposed bases. This forms a new "other half" to each half of the original molecule. After all the bases have new nucleotides bound to them, two identical DNA molecules will be ready for distribution to the two daughter cells. (From Patton KT, Thibodeau GA: *Anatomy and physiology,* ed 7, St Louis, 2010, Mosby.)

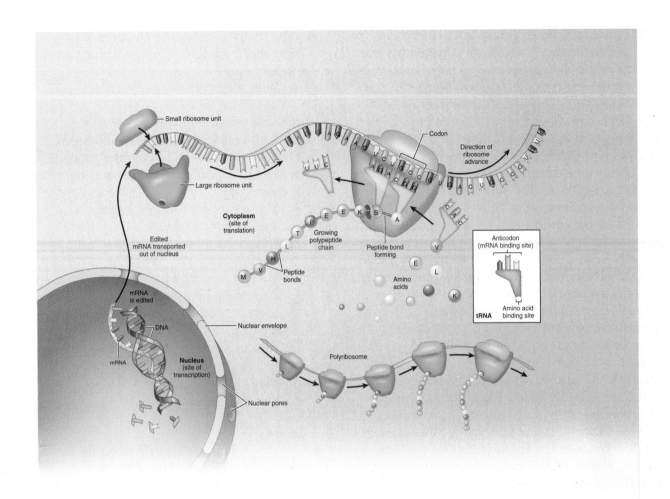

FIGURE 5-12 Protein synthesis begins with *transcription,* a process in which a messenger RNA (mRNA) molecule forms along one gene sequence of a DNA molecule within the cell's nucleus. As it is formed, the mRNA molecule separates from the DNA molecule, is edited, and leaves the nucleus through the large nuclear pores. Outside the nucleus, ribosome subunits attach to the beginning of the mRNA molecule and begin the process of *translation.* In translation, transfer RNA (tRNA) molecules bring specific amino acids—encoded by each mRNA codon—into place at the ribosome site. As the amino acids are brought into the proper sequence, they are joined together by peptide bonds to form long strands called *polypeptides.* Several polypeptide chains may be needed to make a complete protein molecule. (From Patton KT, Thibodeau GA: *Anatomy and physiology,* ed 7, St Louis, 2010, Mosby.)

REVIEW QUESTIONS

1. Why is polarity the most important characteristic of water?
   A. The results of the polarity are hydrogen bonding, a high specific heat value, and its versatile solvent properties.
   B. The results of the polarity are covalent bonding, a low specific heat value, and its versatile solvent properties.
   C. The results of the polarity are ionic bonding, a high specific heat value, and its versatile solvent properties.
   D. The results of the polarity are hydrogen bonding, a low specific heat value, and its versatile solvent properties.

2. Athletes are often concerned with the question of what they need in their diets to increase muscle mass and strength. What biologic molecule would you recommend that would accomplish this?
   A. Carbohydrates
   B. Proteins
   C. Lipids
   D. Nucleic acids

3. Which organelle would you expect to be present in a cell responsible for detoxifying multiple molecules?
   A. Rough endoplasmic reticulum
   B. Smooth endoplasmic reticulum
   C. Lysosome
   D. Golgi apparatus

4. A cell from heart muscle would more than likely contain an unusually high proportion of:
   A. Lysosomes
   B. Mitochondria
   C. mRNA
   D. Ribosomes

5. Which part of cellular respiration produces the greatest amount of ATP?
   A. Electron transport chain
   B. Glycolysis
   C. Krebs cycle
   D. Fermentation

6. When plants do not receive enough water their photosynthetic rated drops. This is because:
   A. Water is a raw material for the light reactions in photosynthesis
   B. Carbon dioxide is not available
   C. Water provides the carbon atoms used to make sugar
   D. Not enough oxygen is produced to keep fermentation running.

7. Which of the following statements is true about the Krebs cycle and the Calvin cycle?
   A. Both result in a net production of ATP and NADH
   B. Both require a net input of ATP
   C. Both result in the release of oxygen
   D. Both use light to initiate the process.

8. Why is it important for cells to undergo mitosis?
   A. Mitosis allows for reproduction with male and female gametes
   B. Mitosis increases variation within the species
   C. Mitosis produces cells that are different from the parent cell
   D. Mitosis produces cells for growth and repair of body tissue

9. 72 Chromosomes undergo meiosis. How many chromosomes will be in each gamete?
   A. 18
   B. 36
   C. 72
   D. 144

10. Which of the following shows how information is transformed to make a protein?
    A. DNA-RNA-protein
    B. Gene-chromosome-protein
    C. ATP-amino acid-protein
    D. RNA-DNA-protein

ANSWERS TO REVIEW QUESTIONS

1. A
2. B
3. B
4. B
5. A

6. A
7. A
8. D
9. B
10. A

CHEMISTRY

C hemistry is a part of our everyday lives. Almost three quarters of the objective information in a client's record consists of laboratory data derived from chemical analytical testing. Laboratory tests and chemical analysis play an important role in the detection, identification, and management of most diseases. The client's evaluation, diagnosis, treatment, care, and prognosis are, at least in part, based on the chemical information from laboratory tests that involve traditional technologies of chemistry. A sound, basic knowledge of chemistry enables the health care professional to reduce the risk of mishandled biologic samples and misdiagnosis and thereby deliver safer and higher quality care.

Chemistry is the study of matter and its properties. Everything in the universe is made or composed of different kinds of matter in one of its three states: solid, liquid, or gas. Matter is defined by its properties. Chemistry is a study of those properties and how those properties relate to one another. Chemistry is a very broad field of study and can be divided into areas of specialization such as physical or general chemistry, biochemistry, and organic and inorganic chemistry. This chapter reviews chemistry from the most basic of substances to complex compounds.

CHAPTER OUTLINE

Scientific Notation, the Metric
    System, and Temperature Scales
Atomic Structure and the Periodic
    Table
Chemical Equations

Reaction Rates, Equilibrium, and
    Reversibility
Solutions and Solution
    Concentrations
Chemical Reactions
Stoichiometry

Oxidation and Reduction
Acids and Bases
Nuclear Chemistry
Biochemistry
Review Questions
Answers to Review Questions

KEY TERMS

Acid
Atom
Atomic Mass
Atomic Number
Base
Basic Unit of Measure
Biochemistry
Catalysts

Celsius
Chemical Equations
Combustion
Compound
Covalent Bond
Decomposition
Deoxyribose
Double Replacement

Electron
Electron Clouds
Equilibrium
Fahrenheit
Groups
Ionic Bond
Isotope
Kelvin

Mathematical Sign	pH	Significand
Mole	Prefix	Single Replacement
Neutron	Products	Solute
Nucleus	Proton	Solution
Orbit	Reactants	Solvent
Periodic Table	Ribose	Synthesis
Periods	Scientific Notation	

Scientific Notation, the Metric System, and Temperature Scales

Scientific Notation

Scientific notation is the scientific system of writing numbers. Scientific notation is a method to write very big or very small numbers easily. Scientific notation is composed of three parts: a **mathematical sign** (+ or −), the **significand**, and the exponential, sometimes called the *logarithm*.

1. The mathematical sign designates whether the number is positive or negative.

> **HESI Hint**
> There is an understood (+) before a positive significand as there is in all positive numbers.

2. The significand is the base value of the number or the value of the number when all the values of ten are removed.
3. The exponential is a multiplier of the significand in powers of ten (Table 6-1). A positive exponential multiplies by factors of ten. A negative exponential multiplies by one tenth (0.1).

> **HESI Hint**
> Some calculators or other devices may write the exponent as an "e" or "E" as in 3.2 e5 or 3.2 E5 instead of 3.2×10^5, which is called E notation.

Example

Consider -9.0462×10^5, where the minus (−) sign means negative, 9.0462 is the significand or base value, and 10^5 is the exponential or multiplier of the significand in the power of ten. In our example above -9.0462×10^5 equals $-9.0462 \times 10 \times 10 \times 10 \times 10 \times 10$ or −904620.

Example

Consider 4.7×10^{-3}, where the absence of the (+) sign is understood as positive, 4.7 is the significand or base value, and 10^{-3} is the exponential or multiplier of the significand in the negative power of ten (as tenths). In our example above, 4.7×10^{-3} equals ($4.7 \times 0.1 \times 0.1 \times 0.1$) or 0.0047.

> **HESI Hint**
> Move the decimal in the significand the number of places equal to the exponent of 10. When the exponent is positive, the decimal is moved to the right and when the exponent is negative, the decimal is moved to the left.

> **HESI Hint**
> When writing a number between −1 and +1 always place a zero (0) to the left of the decimal. Write 0.62 and −0.39 (do not write .62 or −.39); this will avoid mistakes when reading the number and locating the decimal.

Table 6-1 Exponentials*

10^9	1,000,000,000
10^6	1,000,000
10^3	1,000
10^2	100
10^1	10
10^0	1
10^{-2}	0.01
10^{-6}	0.000001
10^{-9}	0.000000001

*1.0 is understood to be the significand with each of the above exponentials.

The Metric System of Measurement

The metric system is a method to measure weight, length, and volume. It is a simple, logical, and efficient measurement system. The basic measurements of the metric system are grams, liters, and meters. A gram (g) is the basic measure of weight, a liter (L) is the basic measure of volume, and a meter (m) is the basic measure of distance.

Each metric measurement is composed of a metric prefix and a basic unit of measure. An example is "kilogram" where "kilo" is the **prefix** and "gram" is the **basic unit of measure.**

The prefixes are the same and have the same meaning or value, regardless of which basic unit of measurement (grams, liters, or meters) is used. Prefixes are the quantifiers of the measurement units. All of the prefixes are based on multiples of ten. Any *one* of the prefixes can be combined with *one* of the basic units of measurement. Some examples are deciliter (dL), kilogram (kg), and millimeter (mm) (Table 6-2) .

Table 6-2 The Prefixes

Prefix	Abbreviation	Means	Numerically
Tera	T-	10^{12}	1 quadrillion times
Giga	G-	10^9	1 billion times
Mega	M-	10^6	1 million times
kilo	k-	10^3	1 thousand times
hecto	h-	10^2	1 hundred times
deka	D-	10^1	10 times
deci	d-	10^{-1}	1 tenth of
centi	c-	10^{-2}	1 hundredth of
milli	m-	10^{-3}	1 thousandth of
micro	μ-	10^{-6}	1 millionth of
nano	n-	10^{-9}	1 billionth of
pico	p-	10^{-12}	1 trillionth of
femto	f-	10^{-15}	1 quadrillionth of

HESI Hint

In medicine, the prefixes in black are the most frequently used (see Table 6-2).

Some comparisons may give more insight to sizes: A meter is a little more than 3 inches longer than a yard. A dime is a little less than 2 cm in diameter. A kilogram is about 2.2 lb. A liter is a little more than a quart.

Temperature Scales

The three most common temperature systems are **Fahrenheit, Celsius,** and **Kelvin.**

Fahrenheit (F) is a temperature measuring system used only in the United States, its territories, Belize, and Jamaica. It is rarely used for any scientific measurements except for body temperature. It has the following characteristics:
   a. Zero degrees (0° F) is the freezing point of sea water or heavy brine at sea level.
   b. 32° F is the freezing point of pure water at sea level.
   c. 212° F is the boiling point of pure water at sea level.
   d. Most people have a body temperature of 98.6° F.

Celsius (C; sometimes called Centigrade) is a temperature system used in the rest of the world and by the scientific community. It has the following characteristics:
   a. Zero degrees (0° C) is the freezing point of pure water at sea level.
   b. 100° C is the boiling point of pure water at sea level.
   c. Most people have a body temperature of 37° C.

Kelvin (K) is used only in the scientific community. Kelvin has the following characteristics:
   a. Zero degrees (0 K) is −273° C and is thought to be the lowest temperature achievable or absolute zero (0).
   b. The freezing point of water is 273 K.
   c. The boiling point of water is 373 K.
   d. Most people have a body temperature of 310 K, but this is never used.

Table 6-3 Important Temperatures in Fahrenheit and Celsius

Condition	Examples of Fahrenheit (F) and Celsius (C) Temperatures	
Melting ice	21° C	32° F
Normal body temperature	37° C	98.6° F
Boiling water	100° C	212° F

Atomic Structure and the Periodic Table

Atomic Structure

The basic building block of all molecules is the atom. An **atom's** physical structure is that of a **nucleus** and **orbits,** sometimes called **electron clouds.** The nucleus is at the center of the atom and is composed of **protons** and **neutrons.** At the outermost part of the atom are the orbits of the **electrons,** which spin around the nucleus at fantastic speeds, forming electron clouds. The speed of the electrons is so great that, in essence, they occupy the space around the nucleus as a cloud rather than as discrete individual locations. The electrons orbit the nucleus at various energy levels called *shells* or *orbits,* almost like the layers of an onion. As each orbital is filled to capacity, atoms begin adding electrons to the next orbit. Atoms are most stable when an orbital is full. However, most of the volume of an atom is empty space. See Figure 6-1 for examples of atoms.

Protons have a positive electrical charge, electrons have a negative charge, and neutrons have

no charge at all. Ground state atoms tend to have equal numbers of protons and electrons, making them electrically neutral. When an atom is electrically charged, it is called an *ion* or it is said to be in an ionic state. This usually occurs when it is in a solution or in the form of a chemical compound. An atom in an ionic state will have lost electrons, resulting in a net positive charge or will have gained electrons, resulting in a net negative charge. The atom is called a *cation* if it has a positive charge and an *anion* if it has a negative charge.

The Periodic Table

Matter is defined by its properties. It can also be stated that the properties of matter come from the properties of their composite elements, and the periodic table organizes the elements based on their structure and thus helps predict the properties of each of the elements (Figure 6-2).

The **periodic table** is made up of a series of rows called **periods** (hence the name periodic table) and columns called **groups.** It is, at its simplest, a table of the known elements arranged according to their properties. It is usually possible to predict, for example, the charge of a main group (the A Group) atom or element, when it exists as an ion, by its location in the table. Group IA has a plus one $(+1)$ charge, group IIA has a positive two $(+2)$ charge, and group IIIA has a positive

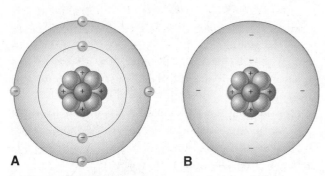

A   **B**

FIGURE 6-1 Models of the atom. The nucleus consists of protons (+) and neutrons at the core. Electrons inhabit outer regions called electron shells or energy levels **(A)** or **(B)** clouds. (From Patton KT, Thibodeau GA: *Anatomy and physiology,* ed 7, St. Louis, 2010, Mosby.)

FIGURE 6-2 Periodic table of elements. (From Patton KT, Thibodeau GA: *Anatomy and physiology,* ed 7, St. Louis, 2010, Mosby.)

3 (+3) charge. Group IVA can have either a positive four (+4) or a negative four (−4) charge. The negative charges are as follows: group VA has a negative three (−3) charge, group VIA has a negative two (−2) charge, and group VIIA has a negative one (−1) charge. Group VIIIA, called the *noble gases*, have no charge when in solution; they remain neutral in nearly all situations. This is because their outer orbits are complete. These gases are also very stable and chemically inert for the same reason. Another property that can be generally deduced by the periodic chart is the number of electrons in the outer electron shell or cloud. Group IA will have one (1) electron in its outer shell. Group IIA will have two (2) electrons in its outer shell. Group IIIA will have three (3), Group IVA will have four (4), and on through all of the A groups. The Groups 3 IIIB through 12 IIB are called *transition metals* and are not as straightforward to predict because of some exceptions to the rules.

HESI Hint

An important principle to remember is that the properties of each element can be predicted based on its location in the periodic chart.

Atomic Number and Atomic Mass

Two important numbers or properties of atoms that can be obtained from the periodic table are the atomic number and the atomic mass.

The **atomic number** is the number of protons in the nucleus, and it defines an atom of a particular element. For instance, any atom that has eleven (11) protons, no matter how many neutrons or electrons, is sodium (Na). If an atom has six (6) protons, it is carbon (C). The atomic number is located at the top of each of the squares in a periodic table. It is always a whole number.

The **atomic mass** of an atom is the *average* mass of each of that element's **isotopes.** Isotopes are different kinds of the same atom that vary in weight. Protons and neutrons each have approximately the same mass or weight, which makes up nearly all of the atom's total mass. The atomic mass is the number at the bottom of each of the squares in the periodic table, and it is usually a decimal number. For a given element, the number of protons remains the same, whereas the number of neutrons varies to make the different isotopes. The most

common isotope of an atom, generally, has the same number of protons and neutrons in its nucleus. The element Carbon 12 (^{12}C), the most common carbon, has (6) protons and six (6) neutrons. The isotope used for "carbon dating" is Carbon 14 (^{14}C), which has 6 protons and 8 neutrons.

Chemical Equations

An element or atom is the simplest form of matter that can naturally exist in nature. It can exist as pure substance or in combination with other elements. When they exist in combination with other elements, the combination is called a **compound,** and they combine in whole number ratios. A part of an element does not naturally exist; at least one atom of the element is present in a chemical reaction. For instance, the elements sodium (Na) and chlorine (Cl) will combine perfectly as whole elements or atoms in a one-to-one ratio to make the compound table salt (NaCl).

Chemical equations are simply recipes. Ingredients, called **reactants,** react to produce a desired end result or compound, called **products.** Equations are written in the following manner:

$$\text{Reactants} \rightarrow \text{Products}$$

In any chemical reaction, an arrow between the reactants and the products is drawn out. This arrow symbolizes the direction of the reaction. Some reactions move toward the product side as seen above, and some reactions will move toward the reactant side with an arrow pointing toward the reactants instead of the products.

$$\text{Reactants} \leftarrow \text{Products}$$

There are also reactions that will create both reactants and products at the same time.

$$\text{Reactants} \leftrightarrow \text{Products}$$

An example is the reaction of aqueous silver nitrate ($AgNO_3$) and aqueous potassium chloride (KCl) to produce solid silver chloride (AgCl) and potassium nitrate (KNO_3).

$$AgNO_3 + KCl \rightarrow AgCl + KNO_3$$

Silver nitrate + Potassium chloride yields
Silver chloride + Potassium nitrate

The law of conservation of mass states that mass cannot be created or destroyed during a chemical reaction. Therefore, once the reactants have been written and the products predicted, the equation must be balanced. The same number of each element must be represented on both sides of the equation. The above example has one silver atom, one nitrogen atom, three oxygen atoms, one potassium atom, and one chloride atom on each side of the equation. Therefore nothing in the way of matter was created or destroyed; it was simply rearranged.

Reaction Rates, Equilibrium, and Reversibility

Chemical reactions generally proceed at a specific rate. Some reactions are fast, and some are slow. A chemical reaction may proceed to completion, but some reactions may stop before all of the reactants are used to make products. These reactions are said to be at **equilibrium.** Equilibrium is a state in which reactants are forming products at the same rate that products are forming reactants. A reaction at equilibrium can be said to be reversible. As the chemicals A and B react to create C and D, C and D react to make more A and B at the same rate.

$$A + B \leftrightarrow C + D$$

Through manipulation of the reaction by various means, shifts in equilibrium, or reversibility, the rate of the reaction can be achieved and controlled. There are basically four ways to increase the reaction rate: increase the temperature in the reaction, increase the surface area of the reactants, add a catalyst, or increase the concentrations of reactants.

Increasing the Temperature

Increasing the temperature causes the particles to have a greater kinetic energy, thereby causing them to move around faster, increasing their chances of contact and the energy with which they collide. Contact is when the chemical reactions will occur.

Increasing the Surface Area

Increasing the surface area of the particles in the reaction gives the particles more opportunity to come into contact with one another. Wood shavings are an excellent example. One can increase the surface area of a log by cutting it into shavings or sawdust. Wood in the form of sawdust will burn or react much faster than a whole log.

Catalysts

A **catalyst** accelerates a reaction by reducing the activation energy or the amount of energy necessary for a reaction to occur. The catalyst is not used up in the reaction and can be collected on completion. Various substances can be catalysts. Common examples include metals and proteins (enzymes).

Increasing the Concentration

Increasing the concentration of the reactants will cause more chance collisions between the reactants and produce more products. Increasing concentration is also a strong determinant of reaction rates. For instance, if there are more cars on the road, there are likely to be more accidents or collisions. The more reactants there are, the faster or more often they will bump into each other and react or become product.

Solutions and Solution Concentrations

Solutions

A **solution** can be defined as a homogeneous mixture of two or more substances. In a solution, there is the **solute,** the part or parts that are being dissolved, and the **solvent,** the part that is doing the dissolving. Solutions can be a liquid in a liquid, a solid in a liquid, or a solid in a solid. The following are types of solutions.

Compounds: Mixtures of different elements to create a single matter.

Alloys: Solid solutions of metals to make a new one such as bronze, which is copper and tin, or steel, which is iron and carbon, tungsten, chromium, and manganese.

Amalgams: A specific type of alloy in which another metal is dissolved in mercury.

Emulsions: Mixtures of matter that readily separate such as water and oil.

Concentration of Solutions—Percent Concentration

Concentration is expressed as weight per weight, as in grams per grams; weight per volume, as in grams per liters; or volume per volume, as in milliliters per liter. Percent concentration is the expression of concentrations as parts per 100 parts. Therefore most concentrations of this type are expressed as milligrams (mg) per 100 milliliters (mL), which can also be written as mg/100 mL or mg/dL. A concentration expression of milliliters (mL) per 100 milliliters (mL) can be written as mL/100 mL or mL/dL.

Concentration of Solutions—Molar Concentration

Molarity, or molar concentration, is a more sophisticated way to express concentrations than is percent. One of the most important concepts in chemistry is the "mole." A **mole** is 6.02×10^{23} of something. This number, 6.02×10^{23}, which is more than a trillion trillions, is known as *Avogadro's number*. A one molar solution will contain 6.02×10^{23} representative molecules of a solute in a liter of solvent. Molar concentrations are written as mol/L. It is important to note that if one measured the atomic mass of any element in grams (g), he or she will have weighed out one mole or 6.02×10^{23} atoms of that element or compound.

Chemical Reactions

A chemical reaction involves making or changing chemical bonds between elements or compounds to create new chemical compounds with different chemical formulas and different chemical properties. There are five main types of chemical reactions: synthesis, decomposition, combustion, single replacement, and double replacement.

Synthesis: In a **synthesis** reaction, two elements combine to form a product. An example is the formation of potassium chloride salt when a solution of potassium (K^+) combines with chloride (Cl^-):

$$2K^+ + 2Cl^- \rightarrow 2KCl$$

Two potassium atoms + two chloride atoms yields 2 molecules of potassium chloride.

Decomposition: **Decomposition** is often described as the opposite of synthesis because it is the breaking of a compound into its component parts.

$$NaCl \rightarrow Na^+ + Cl^-$$

When placed in an aqueous solution, table salt (NaCl) decomposes or breaks apart into an ionic solution of sodium (Na^+) as a cation and chloride (Cl^-) as an anion.

Combustion: **Combustion** is a self-sustaining, exothermic chemical reaction usually initiated by heat acting on oxygen and a fuel compound such as hydrocarbon. In the combustion of hydrocarbon (gas or oil product), the products are carbon dioxide (CO_2) and water (H_2O). The combustion of ethane (C_2H_6) would look like this in a chemical equation:

$$2C_2H_6 \; (g) + 7O_2 \; (g) \rightarrow 4CO_2 \; (g) + 6H_2O \; (g)$$

Ethane + oxygen yields carbon dioxide + water

Single Replacement: Replacement reactions involve ionic compounds; whether the reaction will take place is based on the reactivity of the metals involved. **Single replacement** reactions consist of a more active metal reacting with an ionic compound containing a less active metal to produce a new compound. A good example is the reaction of copper wire (Cu) with aqueous silver nitrate ($AgNO_3$). The copper (Cu) and the silver (Ag) simply swap places. This type of reaction is referred to as single replacement:

$$Cu \; (s) + 2AgNO_3 \; (aq) \rightarrow Cu(NO_3)_2 \; (aq) \\ + 2Ag \; (s)$$

Copper + silver nitrate yields copper nitrate + silver

Double Replacement: **Double replacement** reactions involve two ionic compounds. The positive ion from one compound combines with the negative ion of the other compound. The result is two new ionic compounds that have "switched partners." The example of the reaction of silver nitrate ($AgNO_3$) and potassium chloride (KCl) is a good representation of double replacement:

$$AgNO_3 + KCl \rightarrow AgCl + KNO_3$$

Silver nitrate + potassium chloride yields silver chloride + potassium nitrate

Chemical Bonding

Chemical bonding is the joining of one atom, element, or chemical to another. Some bonds are very weak, and some are nearly unbreakable. In many cases the type of bonding will be determined by the interplay of the electrons in the outer shell of the atom. There are two main types of chemical bonding: ionic and covalent.

Ionic Bonding: An **ionic bond** is an electrostatic attraction between two oppositely charged ions, or a cation and an anion. This type of bond is generally formed between a metal and a nonmetal. An excellent example of ionic bonding is salt. Since opposites attract, the positive cation will attract the negative anion and form an electrostatic bond. In this type of a bond the cation (sodium) takes one electron from the anion (chlorine), which makes the overall molecule electrically neutral.

$$Na^+ + Cl^- \rightarrow NaCl$$

Sodium + chloride yields (table) salt

Covalent Bonding: A **covalent bond** is formed when two atoms *share* electrons, generally in pairs, one from each atom. A single covalent bond is the sharing of one pair of electrons. A double covalent bond is formed when two electron pairs are shared, and a triple covalent bond is formed when three electron pairs are shared. The covalent bond is the strongest of any type of chemical bond and is generally formed between two nonmetals (Figure 6-3).

In a covalently bonded compound, if the electrons in the bond are shared equally, then the bond is termed *nonpolar*. However, not all elements share electrons equally within a bond. When this occurs, a polar bond is the result, which means that the shared electron density of the bond is concentrated around one atom more than the other. Polarity is based on the difference in electronegativity values for the elements involved in

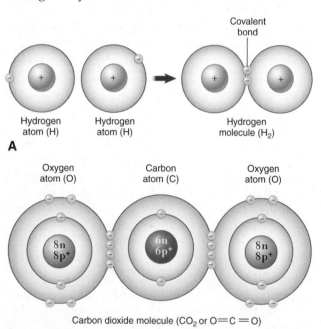

A

B

Carbon dioxide molecule (CO_2 or O=C=O)

FIGURE 6-3 Types of covalent bonds. **A,** A single covalent bond forms by the sharing of one electron pair between two atoms of hydrogen, resulting in a molecule of hydrogen gas. **B,** A double covalent bond (double bond) forms by the sharing of two pairs of electrons between two atoms. In this case, two double bonds form: one between carbon and each of the two oxygen atoms. (From Patton KT, Thibodeau GA: *Anatomy and physiology,* ed 7, St. Louis, 2010, Mosby.)

the bond. The greater the difference, the more polar the bond will be, or one end or side of the molecule will have a charge distinctly more positive and the other side of the molecule will be more negative in charge.

Intermolecular Forces: There are other types of attractions between particles called *intermolecular forces.* These are not bonding interactions between atoms within a molecule but instead are weaker forces of attraction between whole molecules. These forces are hydrogen bonding, dipole-dipole interactions, and dispersion forces.

Hydrogen Bonds: A *hydrogen bond* is the attraction for a hydrogen atom by a highly electronegative element. The elements generally involved are fluorine (F), oxygen (O), and nitrogen (N). Hydrogen bonds are about 5-10% as strong as a covalent bond, making them the strongest of the intermolecular forces.

Dipole-Dipole Interactions: A *dipole-dipole interaction* is the attraction of one dipole on one molecule for the dipole of another molecule. A dipole is created when an electron pair is shared unequally in a covalent bond between two atoms or elements (discussed earlier in polar covalent bonding). Because the electrons are shared unequally, the molecule, not the covalent bond, will have a positive end and a negative end or side. In a solution the molecules will align the charged ends of the molecule north to south or positive to negative, where the north end on one molecule is next to the south end of another. The result is a weak bond between molecules where the more highly electropositive end of a molecule is attracted to the electronegative end of another molecule. This attraction is considered a weak intermolecular force. It is only about 1% as strong as a normal covalent bond.

Dispersion Forces: *Dispersion forces,* sometimes called London dispersion forces, are the weakest of all the intermolecular forces. Sometimes the electrons within an element or compound will concentrate themselves on one side of an atom. This causes a momentary or temporary dipole, which would be attracted to another momentary dipole of opposite charge in another near element or compound.

Stoichiometry

Stoichiometry is the part of chemistry that deals with the quantities and numeric relationships of the participants in a chemical reaction. For a chemical equation to be balanced, numbers called coefficients are placed in front of each compound. These numbers are used in a ratio to compare how much of one substance is needed to react with another in a certain reaction. The process is similar to comparing ingredients in a recipe.

$$2C_2H_6 + 7O^2 \rightarrow 4CO_2 + 6H_2O$$

Ethane + oxygen yields carbon dioxide + water

Using this reaction, determine the number of moles of oxygen that will react with four (4) moles of ethane (C_2H_6). It is possible to determine the number of moles of oxygen needed to complete the reaction by using a process called *dimensional analysis*:

$$\frac{4 \text{ mol } C_2H_6}{} \left| \frac{7 \text{ mol } O_2}{2 \text{ mol } C_2H_6} = 14 \text{ mol } O_2 \right.$$

The ratio of oxygen to ethane is seven to two. By multiplying the given amount of four moles of ethane by the given amount from the coefficient from the equation, one can determine the amount of oxygen needed to react.

Oxidation and Reduction

Oxidation/reduction reactions, called *redox*, involve the transfer of electrons from one element to another. *Oxidation is the loss of electrons, and reduction is the gain of electrons.* It is not possible to have one without the other. The element that is oxidized (loses electron) is the reductant or reducing agent and the element that is reduced (gains electron) is the oxidant or oxidizing agent.

HESI Hint

A good mnemonic is "OIL-RIG" or Oxidation Is Loss, Reduction Is Gain. Think of it this way: to "reduce" an element, one must cause that element's overall electrical charge to become less and that is done by adding or gaining one or more negatively charged electrons (e^-).

A Redox Reaction

Oxidant (gains electron) + e^- $\longleftrightarrow$ Reductant (loses electron) − e^-
        Reduced   Oxidized

The oxidant is reduced because it gains an electron. The reductant is oxidized because it loses an electron.

To identify what has been oxidized and what has been reduced, the oxidation states of all elements in the compound must be determined. The following is a series of rules to make those determinations:

1. The oxidation number of any elemental atom is zero. This means that if an element is in its *natural* state, its number is zero. Most elements in their standard states are single atoms, but a few exceptions exist. Those exceptions are hydrogen (H_2), bromine (Br_2), oxygen (O_2), nitrogen (N_2), iodine (I_2), and fluorine (F_2). These elements, when they exist outside of a compound in their natural state, are always in pairs.
2. The oxidation number of any simple ion is the charge of the ion. If in a reaction, sodium (Na) were listed as an ion (Na^+), it would have an oxidation number of plus one (+1). If chlorine (Cl) were listed as an ion (Cl^-), it would have an oxidation number of minus one (−1).
3. The oxidation number for oxygen in a compound is minus two (−2).
4. The oxidation number for hydrogen in a compound is plus one (+1).
5. The sum of the oxidation numbers equals the charge on the molecules or polyatomic ions.

Example: Assign oxidation numbers to all elements in the following reactions.

$$2C_2H_6 + 7O_2 \rightarrow 4CO_2 + 6H_2O$$

Ethane + oxygen yields carbon dioxide + water

By using the rules listed earlier, we can use simple algebra to solve for the change of electrical charges of those elements not discussed in the rules. Carbon will have to be determined. The first reactant is the compound ethane (C_2H_6). The coefficient of two (2) has nothing to do with the oxidation states of any of the elements and can be ignored. The total charge on the compound is zero, as is determined using rule five. From rule four, hydrogen must have an oxidation state of +1. There are six hydrogen molecules, so the total charge of the hydrogen molecules is +6. Following is the algebra to solve for the oxidation state of carbon (x):

$$2x + 6(+1) = 0$$

Solving for *x*, carbon is found to have a charge of –3.

If the same method is used, the states of all the other elements can be determined. Oxygen in O_2 is zero (rule one). Carbon in CO_2 is +4, and oxygen is −2. Finally, hydrogen in water is +1, and oxygen is −2. With this information, it is possible to predict what is oxidized and what is reduced. Look at the charges on either side of the equation and see what has changed. Carbon goes from a state of −3 to a state of +4. It has lost seven electrons and has therefore been oxidized. Oxygen's state has changed from 0 to −2. It has gained two electrons and has therefore been reduced.

Acids and Bases

Acids are corrosive to metals; they change blue litmus paper red and become less acidic when mixed with bases. **Bases,** also called *alkaline compounds,* are substances that denature proteins, making them feel very slick; they change red litmus paper blue and become less basic when mixed with acids.

Acids are compounds that are hydrogen or proton donors. Hydrogen in its ionic state is simply a proton. In water naked protons exist only for a short time before reacting with other water molecules to produce H_3O^+ a substance called hydronium. Hydronium is a water molecule plus a proton or hydrogen.

Bases are hydrogen or proton acceptors and generally have a hydroxide (OH) group in the makeup of the molecule. This definition explains the dissociation of water into low concentrations of hydronium and hydroxide ions:

$$H_2O + H_2O \leftrightarrow H_3O^+ + OH^-$$

Water + water yields acid + base

In this example, one water (H_2O) molecule acts as a hydrogen donor giving one of its two hydrogens to another water molecule producing the hydronium (H_3O^+) cation and leaving a hydroxyl group (OH). All acids produce hydronium when placed in H_2O. As can be seen, H_2O is amphoteric, which means it can act both as an acid and as a base. In the example above, one molecule of H_2O acts as the proton donor, becoming a hydroxide (OH), and another molecule acts as the proton acceptor, becoming the conjugate acid (H_3O^+).

The concentration of acids is expressed as **pH.** The pH scale commonly in use ranges from 0 to 14 and is a measure of the acidity or alkalinity

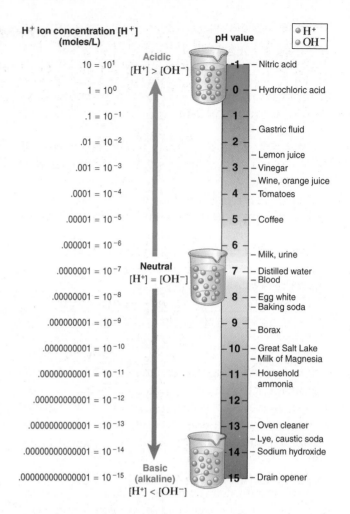

FIGURE 6-4   The pH range. (From Patton KT, Thibodeau GA: *Anatomy and physiology,* ed 7, St. Louis, 2010, Mosby.)

(basicity) of a solution (Figure 6-4). A neutral solution that is neither acidic nor basic has a value of 7. Lower numbers mean more acidic, and higher numbers mean more basic.

Nuclear Chemistry

Chemical and nuclear reactions are quite different. In chemical reactions, atoms are trying to reach stable electron configurations. Nuclear chemistry is concerned with reactions that take place in the nucleus to obtain stable nuclear configurations. *Radioactivity* is the word used to describe the emission of particles and/or energy from an unstable nucleus. The particles and/or energy that are emitted are referred to as *radiation.* The three types of radiation covered in nuclear chemistry are alpha, beta, and gamma.

Alpha radiation is the emission of helium nuclei. These particles contain two protons and two neutrons, causing them to have a charge of plus two (+2). Alpha particles are the largest of the radioactive emissions, and penetration from alpha particles can generally be stopped by a piece of paper.

Beta radiation is a product of the decomposition of a neutron or proton. It is actually composed of high-energy, high-speed electrons that began as neutrons or protons and have "decayed" to electrons. These particles are either negatively charged (electrons) or positively charged (protons). Because they have virtually no mass, beta particles can be stopped by a thin sheet of aluminum foil, Lucite, or plastic.

Gamma radiation is high-energy electromagnetic radiation, similar to x-rays but with more energy. It is very penetrating and can go through several feet of concrete or several inches of lead. Lead shielding is required to block gamma rays.

An isotope is written as an abbreviation with the symbol of the element preceded by a superscript number indicating the atomic mass. For example, Iodine-131 is correctly abbreviated as ^{131}I, and Iodine-125 would be written as ^{125}I. In nature, some isotopes are stable and some isotopes are unstable. Given enough time, unstable nuclei will change or "decay" into more stable forms. The amount of time it takes for half of the unstable isotope in a sample to decay is called the half-life. In nuclear chemistry the atom *decays* until it finds a stable nuclear configuration, usually by emitting radioactive particles. The amount of time used in a half-life (T½) is different for every radioactive element. Some half-lives are very long and some are as short as a few days.

An example of radioactive half-life or decay is ^{131}I, which has a half-life of approximately 8 days, or every 8 days one-half of the radioactive particles will be emitted or decayed. This will happen over and over again until the ^{131}I reaches a stable nuclear configuration.

Biochemistry

Biochemistry is the study of chemical processes in living organisms. Much of biochemistry deals with the structures and functions of cellular components such as carbohydrates, proteins, lipids, and nucleic acids.

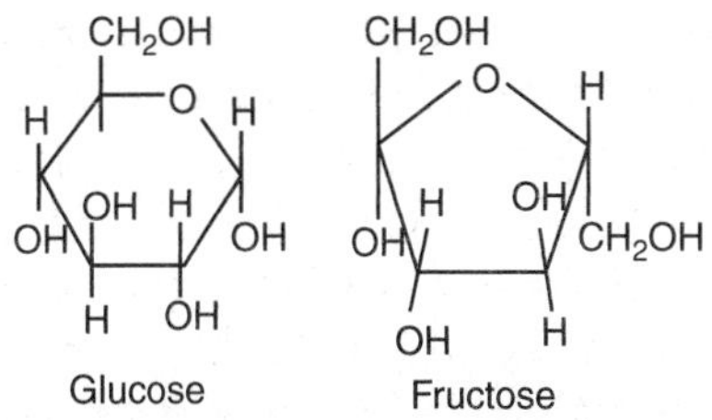

FIGURE 6-5 Molecular configuration for glucose and fructose.

Carbohydrates

Sugars and starches are carbohydrates. Their most important function is to store and provide energy for the body. The sugars **deoxyribose** and **ribose** are used in the formation of deoxyribonucleic acid (DNA) and ribonucleic acid (RNA), respectively. Carbohydrates are more abundant than any other known type of biomolecule.

Monosaccharides The simplest type of carbohydrate is a monosaccharide. Monosaccharides contain carbon, hydrogen, and oxygen, in a ratio of 1:2:1 (general formula $C_m(H_2O)_n$), where m is at least three). Glucose ($C_6H_{12}O_6$) is one of the most important carbohydrates and is an example of a monosaccharide. Fructose ($C_6H_{12}O_6$), the sugar commonly associated with the sweet taste of fruits, is also a monosaccharide. Glucose and fructose are both a six carbon sugar called a *hexose* (Figure 6-5).

HESI Hint

The word "saccharide" comes from a Greek word meaning "sugar."

HESI Hint

Glucose and fructose have the same chemical formula ($C_6H_{12}O_6$) but different actual molecular configurations.

Disaccharides Two monosaccharides can be joined together to make a disaccharide. The most well-known disaccharide is sucrose, which is ordinary sugar. Sucrose consists of a glucose molecule and a fructose molecule joined together. Another disaccharide is lactose, or milk sugar, consisting of a glucose molecule and a galactose molecule. Figure 6-6 illustrates the molecular configuration of sucrose and lactose.

Oligosaccharides and Polysaccharides When three to six monosaccharides are joined together, it is called an *oligosaccharide* (oligo- meaning "few").

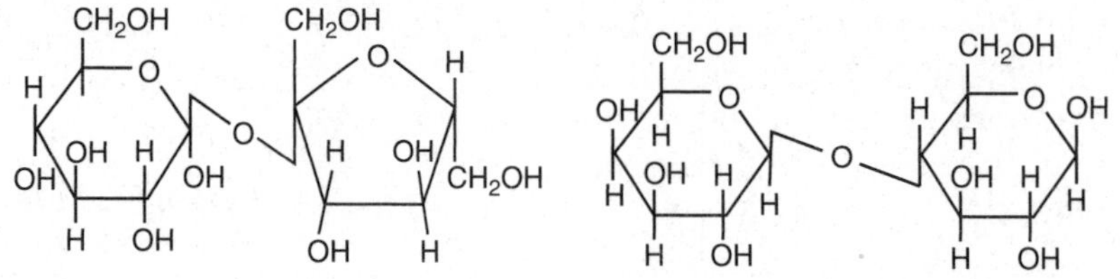

FIGURE 6-6 Molecular configuration for sucrose and lactose.

More than six and up to thousands of monosaccharides joined together make a *polysaccharide*, which can be called a *starch*. Two of the most common polysaccharides are cellulose made by plants and glycogen made by animals, and both of these polysaccharides are chains of repeating glucose units.

Carbohydrates as Energy

Glycolysis Glucose is mainly metabolized by a chemical pathway in the body called glycolysis. The net result is the breakdown of one molecule of glucose into two molecules of pyruvate; this also produces a net two molecules of adenosine triphosphate (ATP). ATP is the substance cells use for energy. In aerobic cells with sufficient oxygen, like most human cells, the pyruvate is further metabolized by a process called *oxidative phosphorylation* (Krebs cycle) generating more molecules of ATP, water, and carbon dioxide. Using oxygen to completely oxidize glucose provides an organism with far more energy than any oxygen-deficient system.

When skeletal muscles are used in vigorous exercise, they will not have enough oxygen to meet their energy demands. They will need to use another type of glucose metabolism called anaerobic glycolysis. Anaerobic means in the absence of or without oxygen. This process converts glucose to lactate instead of pyruvate as in aerobic glycolysis. The production of lactate, an acid, in the muscles creates the "cramp" sensation during intense exercise.

HESI Hint

An aerobic organism or cell requires oxygen to sustain life. An anaerobic organism or cell can function in low concentrations of oxygen, also called micro-aerobic, and some anaerobic organisms exist where no oxygen is present.

Gluconeogenesis The liver can make glucose from other non-carbohydrate sources, such as proteins and parts of fats, using a process called gluconeogenesis. The glucose produced can then enter the energy-producing cycles mentioned previously and undergo glycolysis, or glucose can be stored as glycogen in animals or as cellulose in plants. Glucose can also be used to make other saccharides.

Proteins

Proteins are made up of amino acids. An amino acid is a molecule composed of a carbon atom bonded with four groups: an amine group (NH_2), a carboxyl group (COOH), a hydrogen, and an R group (Figure 6-7). The R group is different for each amino acid, giving each amino acid its own identity and characteristics. Amino acids are joined together to make proteins or parts of proteins. A union of two amino acids using a peptide bond is called a *dipeptide;* a group of less than thirty amino acids are called peptides or polypeptides. Larger groups are proteins. As an example, an important protein in blood called *albumin* contains 585 amino acid residues, and albumin is considered a fairly small protein. In humans, there are only twenty amino acids needed to make all the proteins necessary for life.

Lipids

Lipids are fats and encompass a large group of molecules, including oils, fats, and fatty acids. Fatty acids consist of a hydrocarbon chain with

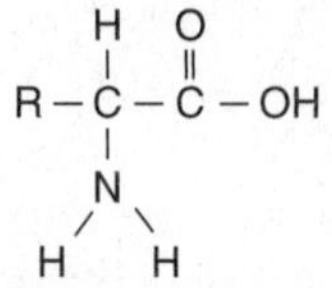

FIGURE 6-7 An amino acid general formula.

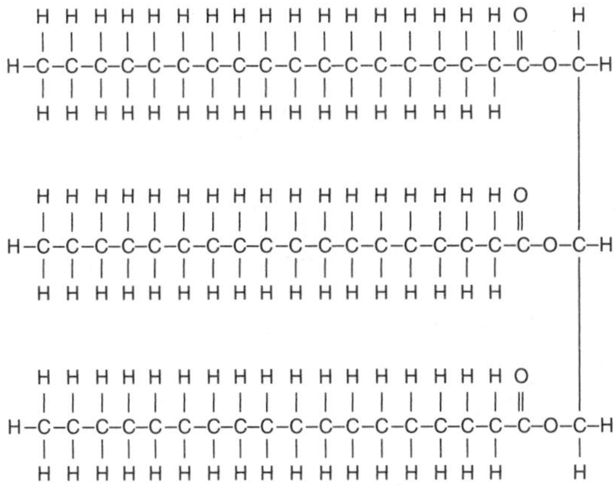

FIGURE 6-8 Three fatty acids attached to a glycerol.

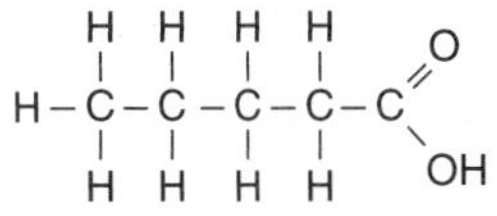

FIGURE 6-9 An example of a saturated fatty acid.

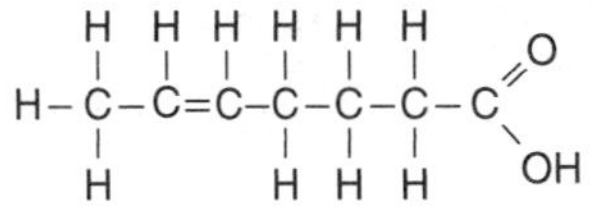

FIGURE 6-10 An example of an unsaturated fatty acid. Note that there are two hydrogens missing, and there is a double bond, designated by two lines, between the two carbons in the center of the fatty acid.

an acid group, the carboxyl group (COOH), at one end. A neutral fat (triglyceride) is three fatty acids generally joined to a glycerol or some other backbone structure (Figure 6-8). Phospholipids are similar to neutral fats but one of the three fatty acids is replaced by a phosphate group. Cholesterol is yet another form of fat composed of a four ring structure and a side chain. Fats are used by the body to insulate body organs against shock, to maintain body temperature, to keep skin and hair healthy, and to promote healthy cell function. Phospholipids are essential components of cell membranes, and cholesterol is an obligatory precursor for many important biologic molecules such as steroid hormones. Fats also serve as energy stores for the body.

Lipids are found in many foods, such as oils, milk, and milk products such as butter and cheese. Natural lipids can be classified as unsaturated, polyunsaturated, and saturated. Saturated fats have no double bond between carbon atoms of the fatty acid chains (Figure 6-9). Unsaturated fats have one or more double bonds between some of the carbon atoms of the fatty acid chains and are more desirable in our diet than saturated fats (Figure 6-10).

Nucleic Acids

Nucleic acids are the biologic brain of life, telling the cell what it will do and how to do it. They include DNA and RNA. Both are nucleotide chains that convey genetic information. Nucleic acids are found in all living cells and viruses. Most nucleic acids are found in the nucleus, but some are found in the cytoplasm and mitochondria of individual cells. They are very large molecules that have two main parts.

The backbone of the molecule DNA is composed of deoxyribose, a five carbon sugar that is also called a pentose, and a phosphate, which alternately chain together in a "sugar-phosphate-sugar-phosphate" chain, making two very long structures. The two chains, or strands, actually twist around each other like the strands of a rope, which is referred to as a "double helix."

The DNA bases adenine, cytosine, guanine, and thymine join the two chains from sugar to sugar much like the rungs of a ladder in a base pair relationship. The pair relationships are constant in that adenine and thymine are always bound together and cytosine and guanine are always bound together in DNA. Note that the two sugar-phosphate chains in DNA run in opposite directions: one up and one down. This is termed *anti-parallel*.

The structure of RNA differs from DNA's structure in that RNA is a single strand of ribose, a five carbon carbohydrate, in a sugar-phosphate chain (Figure 6-11). RNA does not use thymine to form one of its base pairs; it uses instead uracil to bind with adenine. Cytosine and guanine are the other base pair.

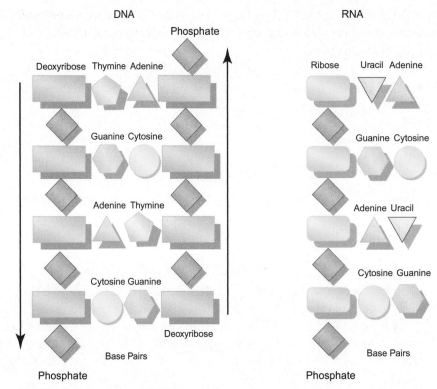

FIGURE 6-11 Structure of DNA and RNA. (Note: The double helix is not illustrated here.)

REVIEW QUESTIONS

1. If an individual weighs 125 lb, what is their weight in kilograms?
   A. 56.8 kg
   B. 2750 kg
   C. 68.5 kg
   D. 100 kg

2. How many protons does potassium (K) have?
   A. 39.08
   B. 32
   C. 19
   D. 13

3. How many neutrons does carbon 14 (^{14}C) have?
   A. 6
   B. 7
   C. 8
   D. 9

4. What would be the oxidation state of the sulfur atom in sulfuric acid, H_2SO_4?
   A. +4
   B. +5
   C. +6
   D. +8

5. What is the strongest type of chemical bond?
   A. Covalent
   B. Hydrogen
   C. Ionic
   D. Dipole interactions

6. Acids are:
   A. Proton acceptors
   B. Proton donors
   C. Electron acceptors
   D. Electron donors

7. When two monosaccharides are joined together they make a:
   A. Polysaccharide
   B. Oligosaccharide
   C. Disaccharide
   D. Fat

8. The nucleic acids DNA and RNA
   A. Are found in the cell nucleus.
   B. Are not found in the cell mitochondria.
   C. Contain different kinds of fat.
   D. Include very small molecules.

9. The reaction $2C_2H_6 (g) + 7O_2 (g) \rightarrow 4CO_2 (g) + 6H_2O (g)$ or ethane + oxygen yields carbon dioxide + water is an example of:
   A. Combustion
   B. Double replacement
   C. Single replacement
   D. Decomposition

10. What is the correct name for $MgSO_4$?
    A. Magnesium sulfate
    B. Manganese
    C. Magnesium sulfite
    D. Manganese silicate

ANSWERS TO REVIEW QUESTIONS

1. A
2. C
3. C
4. C
5. A

6. B
7. C
8. A
9. A
10. A

7 ANATOMY AND PHYSIOLOGY

E very student in the health professions should know the basics of anatomy and physiology. From cells and tissues to organs and systems, the human body is the most complex organism on earth. It is important that members of the health professions who take care of clients know how the human body works as a whole and what role specific parts of the body play in an individual's health and well-being.

A one-year course in anatomy and physiology should be taken before the student prepares for the anatomy examination. Take the time to read about anatomy and physiology at every opportunity. This preparation guide will go through each of the major body systems and point out the most important aspects of facts that should be learned.

CHAPTER OUTLINE

General Terminology	Muscular System	Digestive System
Histology	Nervous System	Urinary System
Mitosis and Meiosis	Endocrine System	Reproductive System
Skin	Circulatory System	Review Questions
Skeletal System	Respiratory System	Answers to Review Questions

KEY TERMS

Alimentary Canal
Anatomic Position
Anterior
Appendicular Skeleton
Arterioles
Axial Skeleton
Bolus
Cell
Cerebellum
Cerebrum
Chyme
Dermis
Distal

Epidermis
Erythrocytes
Estrogen
External Respiration
Hemopoiesis
Histology
Inferior
Infundibulum
Internal Respiration
Lateral
Leukocytes
Medial
Medulla Oblongata

Meiosis
Mitosis
Neuroglia
Osteoblasts
Platelets
Posterior
Progesterone
Proximal
Sarcomeres
Superior
Synergists
Voluntary Muscles

General Terminology

Students of anatomy and physiology should learn the standard terms for body directions and subdivisions of the body. These will provide a basic introduction to the study of the body and also point out the need for the use of correct terminology.

The body planes are imaginary lines used for reference; they include the median plane, the coronal plane, and the transverse plane. A section is a real or imaginary cut made along a plane. A cut along the median plane is a sagittal section. A cut along the coronal plane is a frontal section, and a cut through the transverse plane is a cross-section. When describing the body, visualize the **anatomic position.** The body is erect, the feet are slightly apart, the head is held high, and the palms of the hands are facing forward.

Important terms of direction to review include **superior** (above), **inferior** (below), **anterior** (facing forward), **posterior** (toward the back), **medial** (toward the midline), and **lateral** (away from the midline or toward the sides). **Proximal** and **distal** are terms of direction usually used in reference to limbs. Proximal means closer to the point of attachment, and distal refers to further away from the point of attachment. Figure 7-1 depicts the directional terms.

Major body cavities are divided into the dorsal cavity (includes the cranial and spinal cavities) and the ventral cavity (includes the orbits and the nasal, oral, thoracic, and abdominopelvic cavities).

Additional useful terminology is defined later in this chapter.

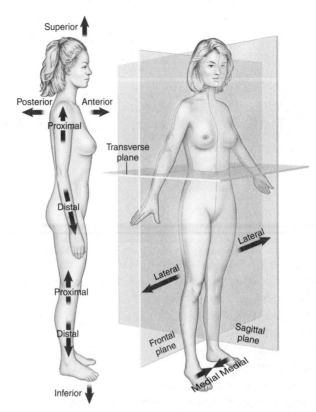

FIGURE 7-1 Planes and directions of the body. (From Patton KT, Thibodeau GA: *Anatomy and physiology*, ed 7, St Louis, 2010, Mosby.)

Histology

Histology is the study of tissues. A tissue is a group of cells that act together to perform specific functions. The four fundamental tissues are epithelial, connective, muscle, and nerve tissues (Figure 7-2). Epithelial cells cover, line, and protect the body and its internal organs. Connective tissue is the framework of the body, providing support and structure for the organs. Nerve tissue is composed of neurons and connective tissue cells that are referred to as **neuroglia.** Muscle tissues have the ability to contract or shorten. Muscle tissue is classified as voluntary muscle (skeletal muscles) or involuntary muscle (smooth muscle and cardiac muscle tissue).

The major parts of the cell should be reviewed. The **cell** is the basic unit of life and the building

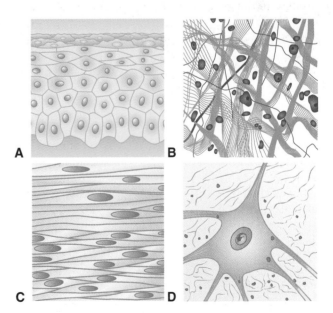

FIGURE 7-2 Major tissues of the body. **A**, Epithelial tissue; **B**, connective tissue; **C**, muscle tissue; **D**, nervous tissue. (From Patton KT, Thibodeau GA: *Anatomy and physiology*, ed 7, St Louis, 2010, Mosby.)

block of tissues and organs. Within the cell, each organelle has a specific function. The nucleus, which contains deoxyribonucleic acid (DNA), and ribosomes are especially important in the synthesis of proteins. Proteins include the enzymes that regulate all chemical reactions within the body.

Mitosis and Meiosis

Mitosis is necessary for growth and repair. In this process, the DNA is duplicated and distributed evenly to two daughter cells. Meiosis is the special cell division that takes place in the gonads, that is, the ovaries and testes. In the process of **meiosis,** the chromosome number is reduced from 46 to 23, so when the egg and the sperm unite in fertilization the zygote will have the correct number of chromosomes.

Skin

The skin is the largest organ of the body. The skin consists of two layers: the **epidermis** (the outermost protective layer of dead keratinized epithelial cells) and the **dermis** (the underlying layer of connective tissue with blood vessels, nerve endings, and the associated skin structures). The dermis rests on the subcutaneous tissue that connects the skin to the superficial muscles.

The layers of the epidermis, from outer layer to inner layer, are the stratum corneum, the stratum lucidum, the stratum granulosum, and the innermost stratum germinativum (includes stratum basale and stratum spinosum), where **mitosis** occurs. Epidermal cells contain the protein pigment called *melanin,* which protects against radiation from the sun.

The inner layer of the skin is the dermis, composed of fibrous connective tissue with blood vessels, sensory nerve endings, hair follicles, and glands. There are two types of sweat glands. The most widely distributed sweat glands regulate body temperature by releasing a watery secretion that evaporates from the surface of the skin. This type of sweat gland is known as eccrine. The other sweat glands, mainly in the armpits and groin area, display apocrine secretion. This secretion contains bits of cytoplasm from the secreting cells. This cell debris attracts bacteria, and the presence of the bacteria on the skin results in body odor. The sebaceous glands release an oily secretion (sebum) through the hair follicles that lubricates the skin and prevents drying. Oil is produced by holocrine secretion, in which whole cells of the gland are part of the secretion. These glands are susceptible to becoming clogged and attracting bacteria, particularly during adolescence.

The appendages of the skin include hair and nails. Both are composed of a strong protein called *keratin.* Skin structure is illustrated in Figure 7-3. Hair, nails, and skin may show changes in disease that may be used in the diagnosis of clinical conditions. For example, skin cancer is a clinical condition that is associated with the skin.

HESI Hint

As the epidermal cells move from the deepest layers to the superficial layers, they move away from their blood and nutrient supply; subsequently, they dehydrate and die. To illustrate this, visualize a large transparent container filled with inflated balloons covered with sticky glue. This illustrates the stratum basale. As the balloons deflate, the sides that are stuck together pull the balloons into a spiny shape, much like the stratum spinosum. As the balloons continue to deflate, they become flattened, like the stratum corneum.

Skeletal System

The body framework consists of bone, cartilage, ligaments, and joints. Functions of the skeletal system include support, movement, blood cell formation **(hemopoiesis),** protection of internal organs, detoxification (removal of poisons), provision for muscle attachment, and mineral storage (particularly calcium and phosphorus).

Individual bones are classified by shape. There are long bones, short bones, flat bones, irregular bones, and sesamoid bones. A typical long bone has an irregular epiphysis at each end, composed mainly of spongy (cancellous) bone, and a shaft or diaphysis, composed mainly of compact bone. The cells that form compact bone are called **osteoblasts;** when they become fixed in the dense bone matrix, they stop dividing but continue to maintain bone tissue as osteocytes.

The **axial skeleton** (Figure 7-4) consists of the 28 bones of the skull. These are separated into the 14 facial bones and the 14 bones of the cranium. The facial bones are two nasal bones, two maxillary bones, two zygomatic bones, one mandible (the only moveable bone of the skull), two palatine bones, one vomer, two lacrimal bones,

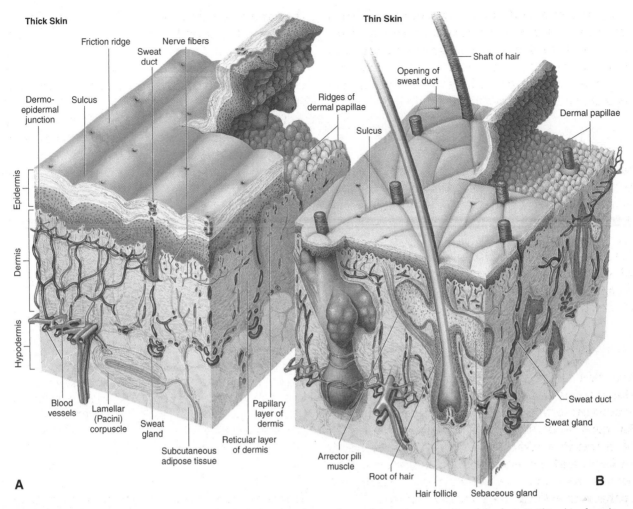

Thick Skin

Friction ridge   Nerve fibers

Sweat duct

Dermo-epidermal junction   Sulcus

Epidermis

Dermis

Hypodermis

Blood vessels   Lamellar (Pacini) corpuscle   Sweat gland

Subcutaneous adipose tissue

Reticular layer of dermis

Papillary layer of dermis

Ridges of dermal papillae

Sulcus

A

Thin Skin

Shaft of hair

Opening of sweat duct

Dermal papillae

Sweat duct

Sweat gland

Arrector pili muscle

Root of hair

Hair follicle   Sebaceous gland

B

FIGURE 7-3 Diagram of skin structure. **A,** Thick skin, found on surfaces of the palms and soles of the feet. **B,** Thin skin, found on most surface areas of the body. In each diagram, the epidermis is raised at one corner to reveal the papillae of the dermis. (From Patton KT, Thibodeau GA: *Anatomy and physiology,* ed 7, St Louis, 2010, Mosby.)

and two inferior nasal conchae. The bones of the cranium are the single occipital, frontal, ethmoid, and sphenoid and the paired parietal, temporal, and ossicles of the ear (malleus, incus, and stapes).

The axial skeleton also has 33 bones of the vertebral column, as depicted in Figure 7-5. There are seven cervical vertebrae, 12 thoracic vertebrae, five lumbar vertebrae, five sacral vertebrae (fused to form the sacrum), and the coccygeal vertebrae (known as the tailbone). The final portion of the axial skeleton consists of the bones of the thorax, the sternum, and the 12 pairs of ribs.

The **appendicular skeleton** (see Figure 7-4) includes the girdles and the limbs. The upper portion consists of the pectoral or shoulder girdle, the clavicle and scapula, and the upper extremity. The bones of the arm are the humerus, the radius and ulna, the carpals (wrist bones),

the metacarpals (bones of the hand), and the phalanges (bones of the fingers). The lower portion of the appendicular skeleton is made up of the pelvic girdle or os coxae. Each of the os coxae consists of a fused ilium, ischium, and pubis. Bones of the lower extremity include the femur (thighbone), the tibia and fibula, the tarsals (ankle bones), the metatarsals (bones of the foot), and the phalanges.

HESI Hint

Construct flash cards for learning the names, locations, and other features of bones and bone markings. Time and practice are more successful learning strategies than trying to "get it" on the first or second time through. Use mnemonic devices to recall the names and positions of bones, foramina, and other anatomic groups within the skeleton.

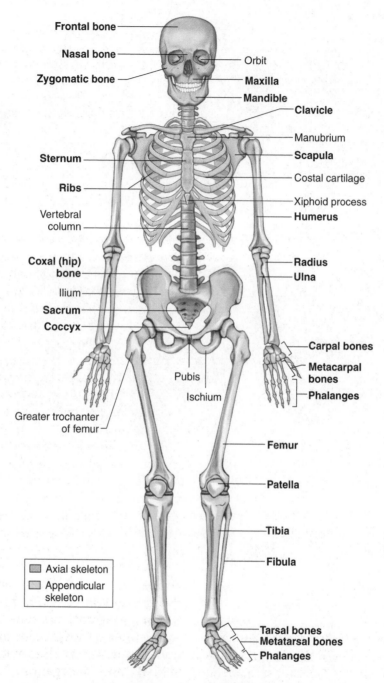

Frontal bone

Nasal bone

Zygomatic bone

Orbit

Maxilla

Mandible

Clavicle

Manubrium

Sternum

Scapula

Ribs

Costal cartilage

Vertebral column

Xiphoid process

Humerus

Coxal (hip) bone

Radius

Ulna

Ilium

Sacrum

Coccyx

Carpal bones

Metacarpal bones

Pubis

Ischium

Phalanges

Greater trochanter of femur

Femur

Patella

Tibia

Fibula

Axial skeleton
Appendicular skeleton

Tarsal bones
Metatarsal bones
Phalanges

FIGURE 7-4 Anterior view of the skeleton. (From Patton KT, Thibodeau GA: *Anatomy and physiology,* ed 7, St Louis, 2010, Mosby.)

Muscular System

Muscles produce movement by contracting in response to nervous stimulation. Muscle contraction results from the sliding together of actin and myosin filaments within the muscle cell or fiber. Each muscle cell consists of myofibrils, which in turn are made up of still smaller units called **sarcomeres.** Calcium and adenosine triphosphate (ATP) must be present for a muscle cell to contract. Nervous stimulation from motor neurons causes the release of calcium ions from the sarcoplasmic reticulum. Calcium ions attach to inhibitory proteins on the actin filaments within the cell, moving them aside so that cross-bridges can form between actin and myosin filaments. Using energy supplied by ATP, the filaments slide together to produce contraction.

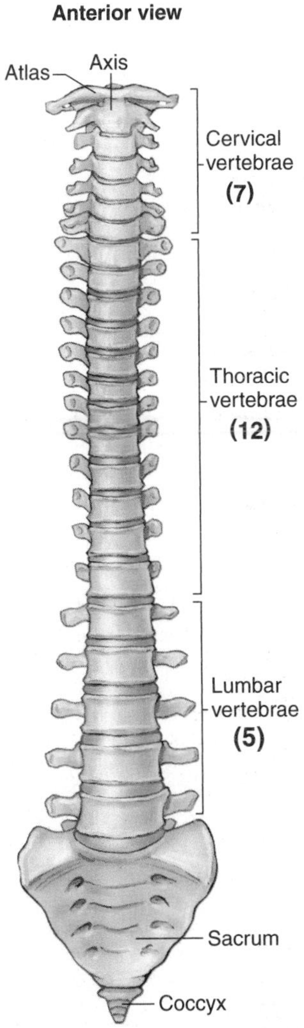

Anterior view

FIGURE 7-5 Anterior view of the vertebral column. (From Patton KT, Thibodeau GA: *Anatomy and physiology*, ed 7, St Louis, 2010, Mosby.)

The skeletal muscles, which make up the muscular system, are also called **voluntary muscles** because they are under conscious control. Skeletal muscles must work in pairs: the muscle that executes a given movement is the prime mover, whereas the muscle that produces the opposite movement is the antagonist. Other muscles known as **synergists** may work in cooperation with the prime mover.

Muscles can be classified according to the movements they elicit. There are flexors and extensors. Flexors reduce the angle at the joint, whereas extensors increase the angle. Abductors draw a limb away from the midline, and adductors return the limb back toward the body (Figure 7-6).

Nervous System

The nervous system consists essentially of the brain, the spinal cord, and the nerves (Figure 7-7). This vital system enables us to perceive many of the changes that take place in our external and internal environments and to respond to those changes (seeing, hearing, tasting, smelling, and touching are examples of perception). It enables us to think, reason, remember, and carry out other abstract activities. It makes body movements by skeletal muscles possible by supplying them with nerve impulses that cause contraction. It works closely with the endocrine glands, correlating and integrating body functions such as digestion and reproduction.

All actions of the nervous system depend on the transmission of nerve impulses over neurons, or nerve cells, the functional units of the nervous system. The main parts of a neuron are the cell body, axon, and dendrites. Dendrites transmit the impulse toward the cell body, and axons transmit the impulse away from the cell body.

The nervous system may be divided structurally into a central nervous system (CNS) and a peripheral nervous system (PNS) (see Figure 7-7). The PNS consists of all the nerves that transmit information to and from the CNS. Sensory (afferent) neurons transmit nerve impulses toward the CNS. Motor (efferent) neurons transmit nerve impulses away from the CNS toward the effector organs such as muscles, glands, and digestive organs.

The major parts of the brain are the **cerebrum** (associated with movement and sensory input), the **cerebellum** (responsible for muscular coordination), and the **medulla oblongata** (controls many vital functions such as respiration and heart rate).

The spinal cord is approximately 18 inches long and extends from the base of the skull (foramen magnum) to the first or second lumbar vertebra (L1 or L2). Thirty-one pairs of spinal nerves exit the spinal cord. Simple (spinal) reflexes are those in which nerve impulses travel through the spinal cord only and do not reach the brain.

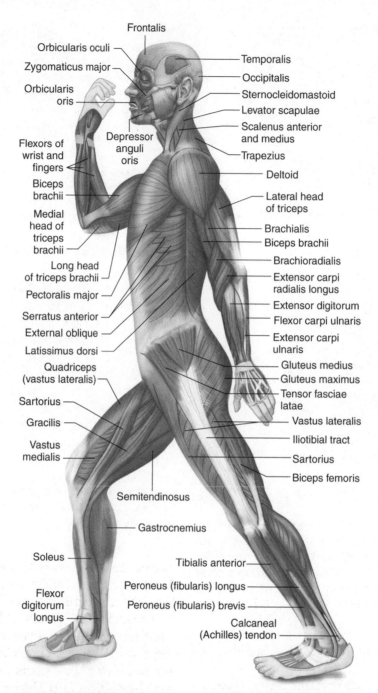

FIGURE 7-6 General overview of the body's musculature (lateral view). (From Patton KT, Thibodeau GA: *Anatomy and physiology*, ed 7, St Louis, 2010, Mosby.)

HESI Hint

Most reflex pathways involve impulses traveling to and from the brain in ascending and descending tracts of the spinal cord. Sensory impulses enter the dorsal horns of the spinal cord, and motor impulses leave through the ventral horns of the spinal cord.

Endocrine System

The endocrine system assists the nervous system in homeostasis and plays important roles in growth and sexual maturation. These two systems meet at the hypothalamus and pituitary gland. The hypothalamus governs the pituitary and is in turn controlled by the feedback of hormones

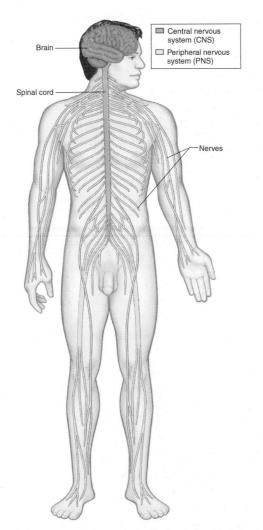

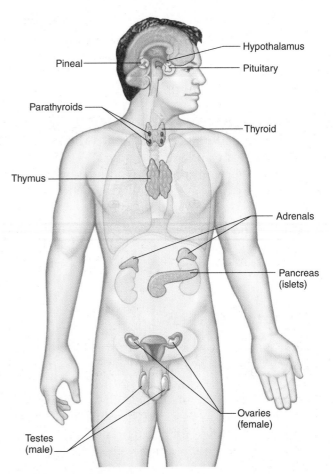

FIGURE 7-8 Locations of some major endocrine glands. (From Patton KT, Thibodeau GA: *Anatomy and physiology*, ed 7, St Louis, 2010, Mosby.)

FIGURE 7-7 Major anatomic features of the nervous system include the brain, the spinal cord, and the individual nerves. The central nervous system (CNS) consists of the brain and spinal cord. The peripheral nervous system (PNS) includes all of the nerves and their branches. (From Patton KT, Thibodeau GA: *Anatomy and physiology*, ed 7, St Louis, 2010, Mosby.)

in the blood. The nervous and endocrine systems coordinate and control the body, but the endocrine system has more long-lasting and widespread effects. Figure 7-8 shows the locations of some major endocrine glands.

Hormones are chemical messengers that control the growth, differentiation, and metabolism of specific target cells. There are two major groups of hormones, steroid and nonsteroid hormones. Steroid hormones enter the target cells and have a direct effect on the DNA of the nucleus. Some nonsteroid hormones are protein hormones. Many protein hormones remain at the cell surface and act through a second messenger, usually a substance called *adenosine monophosphate* (AMP). Most hormones affect cell activity by altering the rate of protein synthesis.

The endocrine glands, although widely distributed, are grouped together as a system because the main function of each gland is the production of hormones. Other organs, such as the stomach, small intestine, and kidneys, produce hormones as well.

HESI Hint

Multiple hormones are released during stress from the adrenal cortex, the hypothalamus, and the posterior and anterior pituitary. The cortisol released from the adrenal cortex reduces inflammation, raises the blood sugar level, and inhibits the release of histamine.

The pituitary gland is nicknamed the master gland. It is attached to the hypothalamus by a stalk called the **infundibulum**. The pituitary gland has two major portions: the anterior lobe (adenohypophysis) and the posterior lobe (neurohypophysis). Hormones of the adenohypophysis are called *tropic hormones* because they act mainly on other endocrine glands. They include the following:

- Somatotropin hormone (STH) or growth hormone (GH)
- Adrenocorticotropic hormone (ACTH)
- Thyroid-stimulating hormone (TSH)
- Follicle-stimulating hormone (FSH)
- Luteinizing hormone (LH)

Hormones released from the posterior lobe of the pituitary include oxytocin (the labor hormone) and antidiuretic hormone (ADH).

Other important endocrine glands include the thyroid, parathyroids, adrenals, pancreas, and gonads (the ovaries and testes).

Circulatory System

Whole blood consists of approximately 55% plasma and 45% formed elements: **erythrocytes** (red blood cells), **leukocytes** (white blood cells), and **platelets.** All of the formed elements are produced from stem cells in red bone marrow. Erythrocytes are modified for transport of oxygen. Most of this oxygen is bound to the pigmented protein hemoglobin. The five types of leukocytes can be distinguished on the basis of size, appearance of the nucleus, staining properties, and presence or absence of visible cytoplasmic granules. White blood cells are active in phagocytosis (neutrophils and monocytes) and antibody formation (lymphocytes). Platelets are active in the process of blood clotting.

Blood serves to transport oxygen and nutrients to body cells and to carry away carbon dioxide and metabolic wastes. Plasma contains approximately 10% proteins, ions, nutrients, waste products, and hormones, which are dissolved or suspended in water.

The heart is a double pump that sends blood to the lungs for oxygenation through the pulmonary circuit and to the remainder of the body through the systemic circuit. Blood is received by the atria and is pumped into circulation by the ventricles. Valves between the atria and ventricles include the tricuspid on the right side of the heart and the bicuspid on the left. Semilunar valves are found at the entrances of the pulmonary trunk and the aorta. Blood is supplied to the heart muscle (the myocardium) by the coronary arteries. Blood drains from the myocardium directly into the right atrium through the coronary sinus.

The heart has an intrinsic beat initiated by the sinoatrial node and transmitted along a conduction system through the myocardium. This wave of electrical activity is what is measured on an electrocardiogram (ECG). The cardiac cycle is the period from the end of one ventricular contraction to the end of the next ventricular contraction. The contraction phase of the cycles is systole; the relaxation phase is diastole.

The vascular system includes arteries that carry blood away from the heart, veins that carry blood toward the heart, and the capillaries. The capillaries are the smallest of vessels and where the exchanges take place between the blood and surrounding tissues, exchanging water, nutrients, and waste products. The systemic arteries begin with the aorta, which sends branches to all parts of the body. As arteries get farther away from the heart, they become thinner and thinner. The smallest arteries are called **arterioles.** The veins parallel the arteries and usually have the same names. The superior and inferior venae cavae are the large veins that empty into the right atrium of the heart.

The walls of the arteries are thick and elastic, and they carry blood under high pressure. Vasoconstriction and vasodilation result from contraction and relaxation of smooth muscle in the arterial walls. These changes influence blood pressure and blood distribution to the tissues. The walls of the veins are thinner and less elastic than those of the arteries, and they carry blood under lower pressure. Figure 7-9 provides an overall view of the circulatory system.

HESI Hint

Deflections of the ECG do not represent the systole and diastole of the heart chambers. Instead, they represent the electrical activity that precedes the contraction-relaxation events of the myocardium. An analogy for this can be at a track meet when the starter's gun is fired before the runners start to run. The sound initiates the action. In the heart, the action potential is similar to firing the gun. The contraction starts just after the action potential passes over the muscle cells.

Respiratory System

Components of the respiratory system include the nose, pharynx, larynx, trachea, bronchi, lungs with their alveoli, diaphragm, and muscles surrounding the ribs. The structural plan of the respiratory system is shown in Figure 7-10. Respiration is controlled by the respiratory control center in the medulla of the brain.

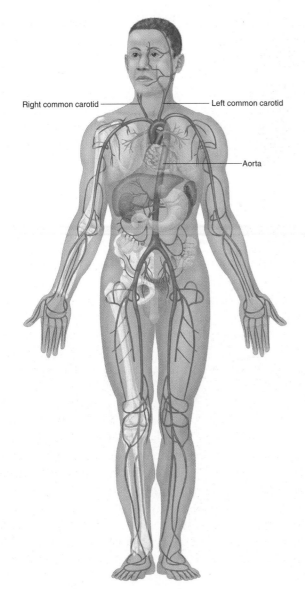

FIGURE 7-9 Principal arteries of the body. (From Patton KT, Thibodeau GA: *Anatomy and physiology*, ed 7, St Louis, 2010, Mosby.)

The respiratory system supplies oxygen to the body and eliminates carbon dioxide. **External respiration** refers to the exchange of gases between the atmosphere and the blood through the alveoli. **Internal respiration** refers to the exchange of gases between the blood and the body cells. The passageways between the nasal cavities and the alveoli conduct gases to and from the lungs. The upper passageways also serve to warm, filter, and moisten incoming air. These upper respiratory tubules are lined with cilia that help to trap debris and keep foreign substances from entering the lungs.

Inhalation requires the contraction of the diaphragm to enlarge the thoracic cavity and draw air into the lungs. Exhalation is a passive process during which the lungs recoil as the respiratory muscles relax and the thorax decreases in size.

Most of the oxygen carried in the blood is bound to hemoglobin in red blood cells. Oxygen is released from hemoglobin as the concentration of oxygen drops in the tissues. Some carbon dioxide is carried in solution or bound to blood proteins, but most is converted to bicarbonate ion by carbonic anhydrase within red blood cells. Because this reaction also releases hydrogen ions, carbon dioxide is a regulator of blood pH.

HESI Hint

Using the familiar example of an inverted tree, you can quickly visualize the trachea as the trunk and the two primary bronchi and their many subdivisions as the branches. The analogy of a bunch of grapes can then be used to explain the terminal components of the respiratory tract, which include the alveolar ducts, alveolar sacs, and alveoli.

Digestive System

The **alimentary canal** or digestive tube consists of the mouth, pharynx, esophagus, stomach, small intestine, large intestine, rectum, and anus. The accessory organs of digestion include the liver, pancreas, and gallbladder. The locations of the digestive organs are seen in Figure 7-11.

Food is ingested into the mouth where it is mechanically broken down by the teeth and tongue in the process of mastication (chewing). Saliva, produced by the three pairs of salivary glands, lubricates and dilutes the chewed food. Saliva contains an enzyme called amylase that starts the digestion of complex carbohydrates. A ball of food called a **bolus** is formed. Constrictive muscles of the pharynx force the food into the upper portion of the esophagus, and the food is swallowed. The esophagus is a narrow tube leading from the pharynx to the stomach. The digestive tract has four main layers, from innermost to outer: the mucous membrane, the submucous layer, the muscular layer, and the serous layer.

Food enters the stomach where gastric glands secrete hydrochloric acid that breaks down foods. The stomach muscle churns and mixes the bolus of food, turning the mass into a soupy substance called **chyme.** The stomach also stores food and regulates the movement of food into the small intestine.

Digestion and absorption of food occurs in the small intestine. Here, food is acted on by various

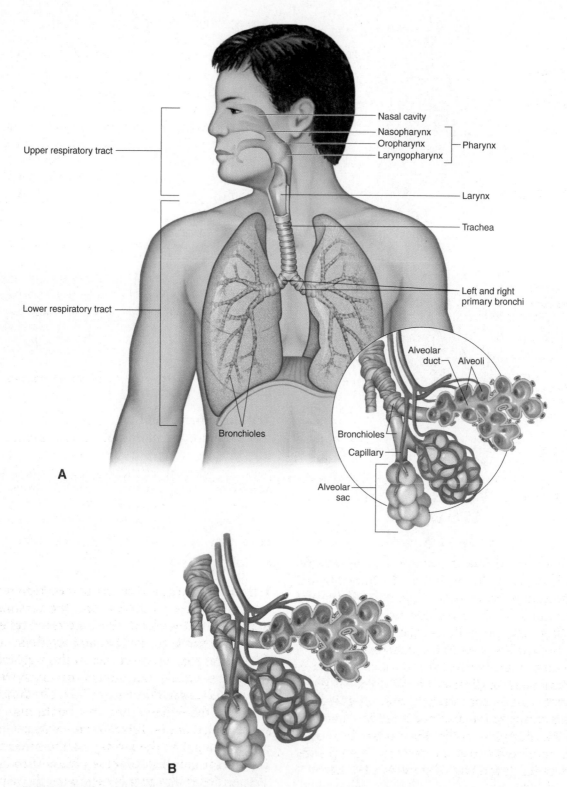

FIGURE 7-10 Structural plan of the respiratory system. The inset shows the alveolar sacs where the interchange of oxygen and carbon dioxide takes place through the walls of the grapelike alveoli. (From Patton KT, Thibodeau GA: *Anatomy and physiology*, ed 7, St Louis, 2010, Mosby.)

enzymes from the small intestine and pancreas and by bile from the liver. The pancreas also contributes water to dilute the chyme and bicarbonate ions to neutralize the acid from the stomach. The small intestine consists of three major regions: the duodenum, the jejunum, and the ileum. Nutrients are absorbed through the walls of the small intestine. The amino acids and simple sugars derived from proteins and carbohydrates are absorbed directly into the blood. Most of the

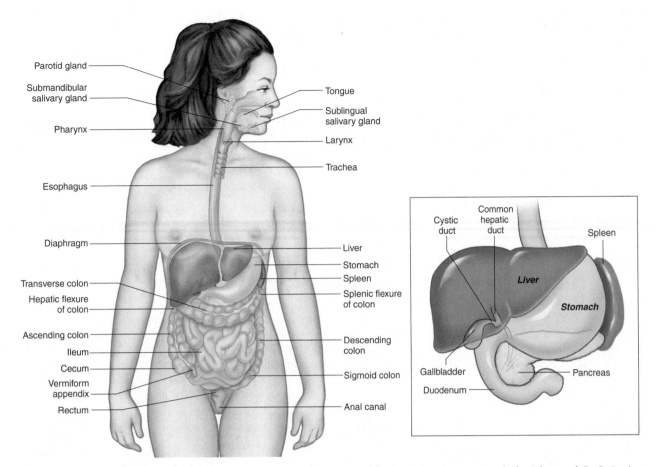

FIGURE 7-11 Location of the digestive organs. (From Patton KT, Thibodeau GA: *Anatomy and physiology*, ed 7, St Louis, 2010, Mosby.)

fats are absorbed into the lymph by the lacteals, which eventually are added to the bloodstream. All nutrients then enter the hepatic portal vein to be routed to the liver for decontamination. Small fingerlike projections called *villi* greatly increase the surface area of the intestinal wall.

The large intestine reabsorbs water and stores and eliminates undigested food. Here also are abundant bacteria, the intestinal flora. The large intestine is arranged into five portions: the ascending colon, the transverse colon, the descending colon, the sigmoid colon, and the rectum. The opening for defecation (expelling of stool) is the anus.

HESI Hint

During mastication, the teeth reduce ingested food material to smaller particles to increase surface area for chemical digestion. Collectively, a bowl of ping-pong balls has far more surface area than a basketball, just as applesauce presents more surface area than a whole apple. The muscular movements of the stomach and intestines also result in mechanical breakdown of food, thus increasing surface area for digestion.

Urinary System

The urinary system consists of two kidneys, two ureters, a urinary bladder, and the urethra. The kidneys filter the blood. The ureters are tubes that transport urine to the urinary bladder, where urine is stored before urination through the urethra to the outside. Location of urinary system organs are illustrated in Figure 7-12. The functional units of the kidney are the nephrons. These small coiled tubes filter waste material out of blood brought to the kidney by the renal artery. The actual filtration process occurs through the glomerulus in Bowman's capsule of the nephron. Filtration of the blood occurs through the glomerulus under the force of blood pressure. As the glomerular filtrate passes through the nephron, components needed by the body, such as water, glucose, and ions, leave the nephron by diffusion and reenter the blood. Water is reabsorbed at the tubules of the nephron. The final product produced by the millions of nephrons per kidney is urine.

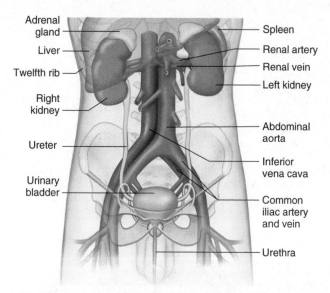

Adrenal gland
Liver
Twelfth rib
Right kidney
Ureter
Urinary bladder

Spleen
Renal artery
Renal vein
Left kidney
Abdominal aorta
Inferior vena cava
Common iliac artery and vein
Urethra

FIGURE 7-12 Anterior view of the urinary organs with the peritoneum and visceral organs removed. (Illustrated by Barbara Cousins in Patton KT, Thibodeau GA: *Anatomy and physiology*, ed 7, St Louis, 2010, Mosby.)

HESI Hint

The analogy of a wastewater treatment facility linked to an incredibly efficient recycling center may help you understand the big picture of urinary system function. The central role of the kidneys is to serve as regulators of our internal environment. Most chemical exchanges with blood occur in the kidneys, where they filter and process the blood to produce urine. In effect, they launder the body fluids of liquid sewage and at the same time retain essential chemicals and nutrients.

Reproductive System

The male and female sex organs (the testes and ovaries) have two functions: production of gametes (sex cells) and production of hormones. These activities are under the control of tropic hormones from the pituitary gland. Reproductive activity is cyclic in women but continuous in men. The gametes are formed by meiosis. Figures 7-13 and 7-14 illustrate the location of male and female reproductive organs.

Male Reproductive System

In men, spermatozoa develop within the seminiferous tubules of each testis. The interstitial cells between the seminiferous tubules produce testosterone. This male hormone influences sperm cell development and also produces the male secondary sex characteristics such as body hair and deep voice. Once produced, the sperm are matured and stored in the epididymis of each testis. During ejaculation the pathway for the sperm includes the vas deferens, ejaculatory duct, and urethra. Along the pathway are glands that produce the transport medium or semen. These include the seminal vesicles, prostate gland, and bulbourethral (Cowper's) glands.

Testicular activity is under the control of two anterior pituitary hormones. FSH regulates sperm production. Interstitial cell–stimulating hormone (ICSH) or LH stimulates the interstitial cells to produce testosterone.

Female Reproductive System

In women, each month, under the influence of FSH, several eggs ripen within the ovarian follicles in the ovary. The **estrogen** produced by the follicle initiates the preparation of the endometrium of the uterus for pregnancy. At approximately day 14 of the cycle, a surge of LH is released from the pituitary, which stimulates ovulation and the conversion of the follicle to the corpus luteum. The corpus luteum secretes the hormones **progesterone** and estrogen, which further stimulates development of the endometrium. If fertilization occurs, the corpus luteum remains functional. If fertilization does not occur, the corpus luteum degenerates and menstruation begins. After ovulation, the egg is swept into the oviduct or fallopian tube. If fertilization occurs, it occurs while the egg is in the oviduct. The fertilized egg or zygote travels to the uterus and implants itself within the endometrium. In the uterus, the developing embryo is nourished by the placenta, which is formed by maternal and embryonic tissues. During pregnancy, hormones from the placenta maintain the endometrium and prepare the breasts for milk production.

HESI Hint

It might be helpful if you think through the processes such as the menstrual cycle. First, learn the functions of each hormone. Then apply them as you move through the cycle. To better remember the cycles and the hormone actions, have a diagram to examine as you go through the cycle.

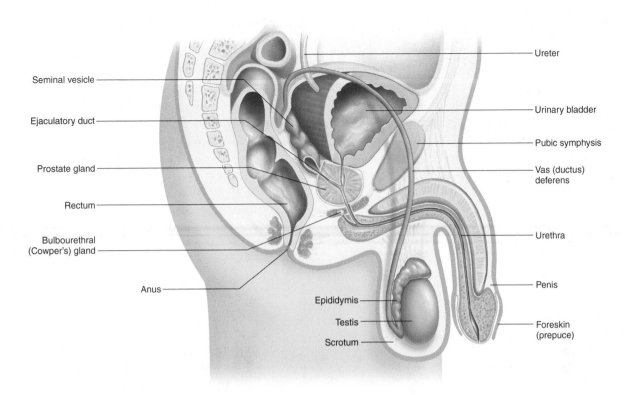

FIGURE 7-13 Male reproductive organs. Sagittal section of inferior abdominopelvic cavity showing placement of male reproductive organs. (From Patton KT, Thibodeau GA: *Anatomy and physiology,* ed 7, St Louis, 2010, Mosby.)

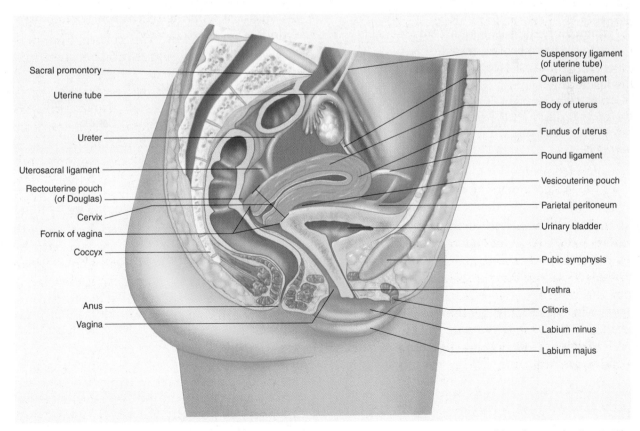

FIGURE 7-14 Female reproductive organs. Diagram (sagittal section) of pelvis showing location of female reproductive organs. (From Patton KT, Thibodeau GA: *Anatomy and physiology,* ed 7, St Louis, 2010, Mosby.)

REVIEW QUESTIONS

1. Which of the following statements is anatomically correct?
   A. The knee is distal to the ankle.
   B. The heart is inferior to the diaphragm.
   C. The hip is proximal to the knee.
   D. The wrist is proximal to the elbow.

2. If you wanted to separate the abdominal cavity from the thoracic cavity, which plane would you use?
   A. Sagittal
   B. Transverse
   C. Frontal
   D. Coronal

3. You have been given a sample of tissue that has pillar-shaped cells arranged tightly together. The tissue you have is:
   A. Squamous epithelium
   B. Cuboidal epithelium
   C. Columnar epithelium
   D. Transitional epithelium

4. The epidermis is classified as a(n):
   A. Cell
   B. Tissue
   C. Organ
   D. System

5. The orthopedic surgeon informs you that you have broken the middle region of the humerus. What area is he describing?
   A. Epiphysis
   B. Articular cartilage
   C. Perichondrium
   D. Diaphysis

6. Going from superior to inferior, the sequence of the vertebral column is:
   A. Sacral, coccyx, thoracic, lumbar, and cervical
   B. Coccyx, sacral, lumbar, thoracic, and cervical
   C. Cervical, lumbar, thoracic, sacral, and coccyx
   D. Cervical, thoracic, lumbar, sacral, and coccyx

7. Which of the following is true of skeletal muscle? (Select all that apply.)
   A. Skeletal muscle comprises 10% of the body's weight.
   B. Skeletal muscle attaches to bones by tendons.
   C. Muscle contraction helps keep the body warm.
   D. Skeletal muscles continuously contract to maintain posture.

8. If an impulse is traveling from a sense receptor toward the spinal cord, it is traveling along what type of neuron?
   A. Motor neuron
   B. Sensory neuron
   C. Interneuron
   D. Bipolar neuron

9. What does the parathyroid hormone regulate?
   A. Magnesium
   B. Calcium
   C. Calcitonin
   D. Glucocorticoids

10. Where are the pressoreceptors and chemoreceptors (specialized sensory nerves that assist with the regulation of circulation and respiration) located?
    A. Circle of Willis
    B. Cerebral arteries
    C. Abdominal aorta
    D. Carotid body

11. Bile is secreted into which organ?
    A. Small intestine
    B. Liver
    C. Large intestine
    D. Stomach

12. What is the role of progesterone in the female reproductive system?
    A. Stimulates ovulation
    B. Conversion of the follicle to the corpus lutem
    C. Stimulates the development of the endometrium
    D. Stimulates the start of the menstruation

ANSWERS TO REVIEW QUESTIONS

1. C
2. B
3. C
4. B
5. D
6. D

7. B, C, D
8. B
9. B
10. D
11. A
12. C

8

PHYSICS

Members of the health professions, particularly medical imaging professionals, use the fundamental principles of physics on a daily basis as they relate to various aspects of imaging science such as radiation safety, radiation dose limits, patient and health professional protection, and patient positioning. Safety and high-quality image production are the goals of all who work within the imaging sciences. Therefore it is essential that students entering the health professions as medical imaging professionals understand the fundamental principles of physics.

The purpose of this chapter is to review the fundamentals of physics relevant to those considering medical imaging careers. In particular, it is a review of the behavior of matter under various conditions and an understanding of basic phenomena in our natural world. Mastery of these basic principles of physics is an integral step toward a career as a health professional in medical imaging.

CHAPTER OUTLINE

Nature of Motion	Uniform Circular Motion	Optics
Acceleration	Kinetic Energy and Potential Energy	Atomic Structure
Projectile Motion	Linear Momentum and Impulse	The Nature of Electricity
Newton's Laws of Motion	Universal Gravitation	Magnetism and Electricity
Friction	Waves and Sound	
Rotation	Light	

KEY TERMS

Acceleration	Joules	Reflection
Average Speed	Kinetic Energy	Refraction
Binding Energy	Law of Universal Gravitation	Scalar Quantity
Centripetal Acceleration	Momentum	Valence Electrons
Force	Newton	Vector Quantity
Friction	Potential Energy	Velocity
Impulse Equation	Projectile Motion	

Nature of Motion

Speed and Velocity

A study of the behavior of matter begins with understanding of the nature of motion. The most fundamental concept to comprehend is average speed. **Average speed** is defined as the distance an object travels divided by the time the object travels without regard to direction of travel. This concept is represented mathematically by the following equation, where v_{av}= average speed, d = distance, and t = time:

$$\text{Average speed } (v_{av}) = \frac{\text{Distance}}{\text{Time}} = \frac{d}{t}$$

SAMPLE PROBLEM

1. A car moves for 10 minutes and travels 5,280 meters. What is the average speed of the car?
   A. 528 m/sec
   B. 52.8 m/sec
   C. 8.8 m/sec
   D. 88 m/sec

Answer

C—Average speed is the distance an object travels divided by the time the object travels. First, the answers must be expressed in m/sec; therefore the time of travel by the car must be converted from minutes to seconds before the average speed is determined:

$$\frac{x}{10 \text{ min}} = \frac{60 \text{ sec}}{1 \text{ min}}$$

$$x = \frac{60 \text{ sec} \times 10 \text{ min}}{1 \text{ min}}$$

$$x = 600 \text{ sec}$$

Dividing the distance traveled by the car (5,280 meters) by the new value for time traveled by the car (600 seconds) determines that the average speed of the car is 8.8 m/sec.

$$\text{Average speed } (v_{av}) = \frac{\text{Distance}}{\text{Time}}$$

$$\text{Average speed} = \frac{5280 \text{ m}}{600 \text{ sec}}$$

$$\text{Average speed} = 8.8 \text{ m/sec}$$

An important related concept is velocity. **Velocity** refers to speed in a specific direction.

Speed is a **scalar quantity** (quantity described simply by a numeric value) and is expressed in units of magnitude. Velocity is a **vector quantity** (quantity describing the time rate of change of an object's position) and must be expressed in both units of magnitude (i.e., speed) and direction of motion.

The average velocity of an object is determined by averaging the initial speed and the final speed of the object (add the two together and divide by 2). This concept is represented mathematically by the following equation, where v_f = final velocity and v_i = initial velocity.

$$v_{av} = \frac{v_f + v_i}{2}$$

Acceleration

Often, objects in motion change velocity over a period of time. Such a change in motion is called **acceleration** and is defined as the rate of change in velocity over a period of time. Acceleration is a vector quantity and is expressed in terms of magnitude and direction. This concept is represented mathematically by the following equation, where a = acceleration, v_f = final velocity, v_i = initial velocity, and Δt = the change in time.

$$\text{Acceleration}(a) = \frac{\Delta \text{ Velocity}}{\Delta \text{ Time}} = \frac{\Delta v}{\Delta t} = \frac{v_f - v_i}{\Delta t}$$

SAMPLE PROBLEM

2. A cart is set in motion. The cart has an initial speed of 15 m/sec and moves for 25 seconds. At the end of 25 seconds, the cart's speed is 40 m/sec. What is the magnitude of the cart's acceleration?
   A. 1.0 m/sec^2
   B. 2.2 m/sec^2
   C. 10.0 m/sec^2
   D. 1.1 m/sec^2

Answer

A—Acceleration is determined by dividing the change in the cart's velocity (final velocity [40 m/sec] – initial velocity [15 m/sec] = 25 m/sec) by the length of time the cart was in motion (25 seconds), indicating the cart is accelerating at 1.0 m/sec^2.

$$\text{Acceleration}(a) = \frac{v_f - v_i}{\Delta t}$$

$$a = \frac{40 \text{ m/sec} - 15 \text{ m/sec}}{25 \text{ sec}}$$

$$a = \frac{25 \text{ m/sec}}{25 \text{ sec}}$$

$$a = 1.0 \text{ m/sec}^2$$

Projectile Motion

The acceleration of objects released above the surface of the earth is influenced by the force of gravity. Gravity, assuming no wind resistance, accelerates an object released above the earth's surface at a rate of 9.8 m/sec². For example, if a rock is released from rest and falls toward the earth, the speed of the rock will increase by 9.8 m/sec for every second the object falls. At the end of 3 seconds the object will have a speed of 29.4 m/sec and a velocity of 29.4 m/sec in the direction toward Earth's surface.

It is also possible for an object to display two types of motion simultaneously. This motion is generally called **projectile motion**. If a can is kicked from the edge of a cliff, the can will move horizontally at the same time it falls toward Earth (Figure 8-1). The horizontal motion is not an accelerated motion; therefore horizontal distance (d_x) is a function of velocity (v_x) and time *(t)* based on the following mathematic expression, where the x subscript is used to denote motion along the horizontal plane (x axis).

$$d_x = v_x t$$

The vertical motion is more complicated. Gravity is acting vertically, so the velocity along the vertical plane (y axis) is constantly changing. The following mathematic expressions represent several methods of describing vertical motion, where v_f = final velocity, v_i = initial velocity, a = acceleration, d = distance, and t = time.

$$v_f^2 = v_i^2 + 2ad$$
$$d = \tfrac{1}{2}at^2 + v_i t$$
$$v_f = v_i + at$$

SAMPLE PROBLEM

3. A can is kicked off a cliff that is 19.6 m tall. The horizontal speed given to the can is 12.0 m/sec. Assuming there is no air resistance, how far out from the base of the cliff will the can land?
    A. 12.0 m
    B. 39.2 m
    C. 6.0 m
    D. 24.0 m

Answer

D—The problem provides values for the vertical distance (height of cliff), vertical acceleration (gravitational constant), and the initial vertical velocity (at rest on cliff, thus 0). The first step is to calculate time of flight. The following equation can be transformed to determine the time of flight.

$$d = \tfrac{1}{2}at^2 + v_i t$$

$v_i t$ drops out of the equation because the initial vertical velocity is 0.

$$d = \tfrac{1}{2}at^2$$

Convert the equation to solve for time.

$$t = \sqrt{\frac{d}{\tfrac{1}{2}a}}$$

$$t = \sqrt{\frac{19.6 \text{ m}}{\tfrac{1}{2}(9.8 \text{ m/sec}^2)}}$$

$$t = 2.0 \text{ sec}$$

Once the time of flight is determined, insert the appropriate values into the horizontal distance equation to solve for horizontal distance.

$$d_x = v_x t$$
$$d_x = 12 \text{ m/sec} \times 2 \text{ sec}$$
$$d_x = 24 \text{ m}$$

Assuming no air resistance, the can will land 24.0 m from the cliff.

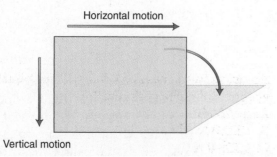

Horizontal motion

Vertical motion

FIGURE 8-1   Projectile motion.

Newton's Laws of Motion

Before delving into Newton's laws of motion, a brief discussion of force is necessary. **Force** is defined as a push or pull on an object. When two forces are equal in magnitude and in opposing directions, they cancel each other out and result in a balanced force. However, if one of the two forces is greater than the other, then an unbalanced force exists and with it acceleration. Net force is simply the sum of the individual forces acting on an object. Keep in mind that the + and − signs are used to indicate direction of force and the mathematic rules associated with summing negative and positive numbers apply.

Newton's First Law of Motion

Newton's first law of motion states that a body at rest will remain at rest, and a body in motion will remain in motion with a constant velocity, unless acted on by an unbalanced force (a force not opposed by one of equal magnitude and in the opposite direction). Newton's second law of motion states that an unbalanced force will cause acceleration, and this acceleration is directly proportional to the unbalanced force. This relationship is expressed mathematically as follows, where F = force, a = acceleration, and k = the constant of proportionality.

$$F = ka$$

Newton's Second Law of Motion

When used in Newton's second law of motion, the constant of proportionality (k) is equal to the mass of the object. Therefore Newton's second law is expressed mathematically as follows, where F = force, m = mass, and a = acceleration.

$$F = ma$$

SAMPLE PROBLEM

4. A box rests on a tabletop. The box has a mass of 25 kg and is acted on by two forces. The force pushing to the right is 96 N, whereas the force pushing to the left is 180 N. Determine the magnitude of the acceleration of the box.
   A. 11.0 m/sec^2
   B. 3.4 m/sec^2
   C. 5.5 m/sec^2
   D. 7.2 m/sec^2

Answer

B—To determine the acceleration of the box, it is necessary to first determine the net force acting on the box. Remember that the net force acting on the box is simply the sum of all forces acting on the box. Because the two forces are opposing each other, one force is considered a positive force and the other a negative force. Therefore net force is represented by the following mathematic equation and is determined to be 84 N to the left.

$$\text{NetForce} = F_{\text{left}} + (-)\, F_{\text{right}}$$
$$\text{NetForce} = 180\,\text{N} + (-)\, 96\,\text{N}$$
$$\text{NetForce} = 84\,\text{N} \leftarrow$$

Once the net force is determined, use Newton's second law equation to determine the magnitude of acceleration of the box.

$$F = ma$$

First, convert the formula to solve for acceleration.

$$a = \frac{F}{m}$$

$$a = \frac{84\,\text{N}}{25\,\text{kg}}$$

The acceleration of the box is determined to be 3.4 m/sec^2. NOTE: Newtons are also expressed in kg-m/sec^2.

If the mass is expressed in kilograms and the acceleration is expressed in meters per second squared (m/sec^2), the unit of force is referred to as the **newton** (N) and is equal to the force necessary to accelerate a mass of one kilogram one meter per second per second. Weight is simply a specialized case of Newton's second law. Weight can be stated mathematically as follows, where m = mass in kilograms and g = 9.8 m/sec^2 (i.e., the rate of acceleration associated with gravity).

$$W = mg$$

SAMPLE PROBLEM

5. An object has a mass of 1,250 g. Determine the weight of the object on Earth.
   A. 12,250 N
   B. 122.50 N
   C. 1,225.0 N
   D. 12.25 N

Answer

D—To determine the weight of the object on Earth, first convert the units of mass to kilograms (1,250 g = 1.25 kg). Second, insert the appropriate values into the weight equation.

$$W = mg$$
$$W = 1.25 \, \text{kg} \times 9.8 \, \text{m/sec}^2$$
$$W = 12.25 \, \text{N}$$

The weight of the object on Earth is determined to be 12.25 N.

Newton's Third Law of Motion

Newton's third law of motion states that for every action there must be an equal and opposite reaction.

Friction

Friction is a force that opposes motion and is expressed in newtons. If a box (Figure 8-2) is slid on a surface at a constant rate by an applied force, we can deduce that friction is present and is opposing the motion of the box. Because there is no acceleration of the box, it is clear that friction is present and all forces are balanced. This relationship of balanced forces is represented in the diagram. Note that the normal force *(A)* and the weight *(B)* are balanced. The applied force *(C)* is to the right and has a magnitude of 100 N. The frictional force *(D)* is to the left and must also be 100 N if the box has no acceleration.

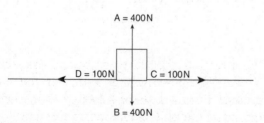

FIGURE 8-2 Depiction of a box being slid on a surface at a constant rate by an applied force.

6. A crate is pulled to the right by a rope attached to the crate. The force applied to the rope is 600 N. As the crate slides along the floor, there is a frictional force between the crate and the floor that has a magnitude of 450 N. Determine the magnitude of the net force acting on the crate.
   A. 1,050 N
   B. 600 N
   C. 150 N
   D. 450 N

Answer

C—To determine the magnitude of the net force acting on the crate, remember that the magnitude of the net force acting on the box is simply the sum of all forces acting on the box. Because the two forces are opposing each other, applied force to the right and friction to the left, the magnitude of the net force is represented by the following mathematic equation and is determined to be 150 N to the right.

$$\text{NetForce} = F_{\text{right}} + (-) \, F_{\text{left}}$$
$$\text{NetForce} = 600 \, \text{N} + (-)450 \, \text{N}$$
$$\text{NetForce} = 150 \, \text{N} \rightarrow$$

Rotation

In addition to displaying linear motion, an object may display a rotating or circular motion. The relationship between the angular displacement and the radius of the circle is expressed mathematically as follows, where θ = the angular displacement, s = arc length, and r = radius of the circle through which the object is moving.

$$\theta = \frac{s}{r}$$

The average speed of the circular motion can be described by looking at the number of rotations or revolutions an object makes in a given time. The angular speed is the number of radians completed in a given time unit. This is expressed mathematically as follows, where ω = angular speed, θ = the angular displacement, and t = time. When the mathematic expression is considered, it is important to remember that there are 2π radians in one revolution.

$$\omega = \frac{\Delta\theta}{\Delta t}$$

It is also possible to have an angular acceleration as a spinning or rotating object gains or loses speed. This is expressed mathematically as follows, where α = angular acceleration, ω = angular speed, and t = time.

$$\alpha = \frac{\Delta\omega}{\Delta t}$$

The relationship between linear motion and rotational motion is analogous and conforms to Newton's laws. Box 8-1 provides a description of the relationship between the mathematic expressions describing linear motion and those describing rotational motion. Beside each linear motion formula is its rotational motion counterpart. The expressions have been defined and applied within this chapter.

Box 8-1 Mathematic Expressions Describing Linear and Rotational Motion

Linear Motion	Rotational Motion
$d = v_{av}t$	$\theta = \omega_{av}t$
$v_f = v_i + at$	$\omega_f = \omega_i + \alpha t$
$d = \frac{1}{2}at^2 + v_i t$	$\theta = \frac{1}{2}\alpha t^2 + \omega_i t$
$v_f^2 = v_i^2 + 2ad$	$\omega_f^2 = \omega_i^2 + 2\alpha\theta$

SAMPLE PROBLEM

7. If a bicycle wheel goes from 48 revolutions per second to 84 revolutions per second in 11 seconds, what is the angular acceleration of the wheel?
   A. 3.27 revolutions/sec^2
   B. 6.00 revolutions/sec^2
   C. 12.0 revolutions/sec^2
   D. 1.64 revolutions/sec^2

Answer

A—To determine the angular acceleration, divide the change in angular speed by the time it took to complete the change in speed.

$$\omega_f = \omega_i + \alpha t$$

Convert the equation to solve for angular acceleration (*a*).

$$\alpha = \frac{\omega_f - \omega_i}{t}$$

$$\alpha = \frac{84 \text{ rev/sec} - 48 \text{ rev/sec}}{11 \text{ sec}}$$

$$\alpha = 3.27 \text{ rev/sec}^2$$

Uniform Circular Motion

It is possible for an object to experience acceleration even though the object is moving at a constant speed. This is possible because acceleration is a vector quantity and is defined as a change in velocity over a change in time. Velocity has a magnitude and a direction, so even though the speed or magnitude of the velocity is constant, the direction could be changing. In uniform circular motion, this is exactly what is happening. Therefore the object is undergoing an acceleration called a **centripetal acceleration** (rotational motion equivalent of acceleration). Centripetal acceleration is represented mathematically as follows, where a_c = centripetal acceleration, v = the speed of the object in meters per second, and r = the radius of the circle.

$$a_c = \frac{v^2}{r}$$

Because there is a centripetal acceleration, there must also be a centripetal force. Newton's law states that force is a function of mass and acceleration; therefore centripetal force must be a function of mass of an object and centripetal acceleration. This relationship is expressed mathematically as follows, where F_c = centripetal force, m = the mass of the object, v = the velocity, and r = the radius of the circle.

$$F_c = \frac{mv^2}{r}$$

The direction of both the force and the acceleration must be toward the center of the circle. Think of whirling a stone attached to a string in a horizontal circle. The tension in the cord keeps the stone moving in a circular path by pulling inward on the stone.

8. A 0.6-kg rock is spun in a circle on a 1.2-m string. If the string breaks at 15 N of tension, how fast must the rock be moving?
   A. 30 m/sec
   B. 6 m/sec
   C. 5 m/sec
   D. 5.5 m/sec

Answer
D—The centripetal force (15 N) is supplied by the tension in the string. The radius of the circle is 1.2 m, and the mass of the rock is 0.6 kg. After these values are inserted in the centripetal force equation, the speed of the stone is determined to be 5.5 m/sec.

$$F_c = \frac{mv^2}{r}$$

Convert the equation to solve for velocity.

$$v = \sqrt{\frac{F_c r}{m}}$$

$$v = \sqrt{\frac{(15\text{ N})(1.2\text{ m})}{0.6\text{ kg}}}$$

$$v = 5.5\text{ m/sec}$$

Kinetic Energy and Potential Energy

Kinetic energy of an object is the energy resulting from the motion of the object and is represented by the following equation, where KE = kinetic energy, m = mass of the object, and v = velocity.

$$KE = \tfrac{1}{2}mv^2$$

In this equation, mass must be expressed in kilograms and velocity must be expressed in meters per second.

The **potential energy** of an object is the energy the object has because of its position and is expressed by the following equation, where PE = potential energy, m = mass of the object, g = acceleration caused by gravity, and h = the height at which the object is located above the ground.

$$PE = mgh$$

In this equation, mass must be expressed in kilograms, gravity is a constant expressed as 9.8 m/sec², and height is expressed in meters.

Kinetic energy, and potential energy are scalar quantities and are expressed in units called **joules**. A joule is a newton-meter or a kilogram-meter squared per second squared (kg-m²/sec²). Remember that the law of conservation of energy states that energy must be conserved; therefore kinetic energy and potential energy can be interchanged if we assume that there is no friction or air resistance present.

9. A car has a mass of 1,100 kg and is moving at 24 m/sec. How much kinetic energy does the car have as a result of its motion?
   A. 26,400 J
   B. 13,200 J
   C. 633,600 J
   D. 316,800 J

Answer
D—The problem provides values for mass and velocity; after the appropriate values for kinetic energy are inserted into the equation, the kinetic energy as a result of the car's motion is determined to be 316,800 J.

$$KE = \tfrac{1}{2}mv^2$$

$$KE = \tfrac{1}{2}(1,100\text{ kg})(24\text{ m/sec})^2$$

$$KE = 316,800\text{ J}$$

Linear Momentum and Impulse

Considering Newton's second law of motion in the following slightly different form allows for the development of a new relationship.

$$F = \frac{m\Delta v}{\Delta t}$$

If both sides of this equation are multiplied by Δt, a new relationship between force and time is established and expressed as follows:

$$F\Delta t = m\Delta v$$

The new relationship is referred to as the **impulse equation** because a force applied over a period of time is an impulse. This impulse causes a change in velocity of the object, which results in a change in momentum of the object. **Momentum** is defined as the amount of motion displayed by an object and is represented by the following mathematical equation, where p = the momentum in kilograms-meters per second, m = the mass in kilograms, and Δv = the change in velocity of the object.

$$p = m\Delta v$$

Momentum is a vector quantity, which means we must have both magnitude and direction to completely express momentum. Momentum must always be conserved, so the momentum before an interaction must equal the momentum after an interaction. This relationship is expressed mathematically as follows, where m_1 and m_2 = masses 1 and 2, v_1' and v_2' = the initial velocities of objects 1 and 2, and v_1 and v_2 = the final velocities of objects 1 and 2 after the interaction.

$$m_1v_1' + m_2v_2' = m_1v_1 + m_2v_2$$

SAMPLE PROBLEM

10. A 30-g rubber ball traveling at 1.60 m/sec strikes a motionless 400-g block of wood. If the ball bounces backward off the block of wood at 1.00 m/sec, how fast will the block of wood be moving?
    A. 0.045 m/sec
    B. 0.195 m/sec
    C. 0.60 m/sec
    D. 1.00 m/sec

Answer
A—With the conservation of momentum equation, with the rubber ball established as mass 1 and the block of wood as mass 2, and with the initial velocity of the block of wood being 0, the speed of the block of wood after impact with the ball is determined to be 0.045 m/sec.

$$m_1v_1 + m_2v_2 = m_1v_1' + m_2v_2'$$

Convert the equation to solve for the speed of the block after impact (v_2').

$$v_2' = \frac{m_1v_1 + m_2v_2 - m_1v_1'}{m_2}$$

$$v_2' = \frac{(30 \text{ g} \times 1.60 \text{ m/sec}) + (400 \text{ g} \times 1.60 \text{ m/sec}) - (30 \text{ g} \times 1.0 \text{ m/sec})}{400 \text{ g}}$$

$$v_2' = 0.045 \text{ m/sec}$$

Universal Gravitation

Newton stated that every object in the universe attracts every other object in the universe. This statement is known as the **law of universal gravitation** and is expressed mathematically as follows, where F = force of attraction, m_1 and m_2 = the masses of objects 1 and 2 expressed in kilograms, G = the universal gravitation constant ($6.67 \times 10^{-11} \text{ Nm}^2/\text{kg}^2$), and r = the distance between the two objects expressed in meters.

$$F = \frac{Gm_1 m_2}{r^2}$$

SAMPLE PROBLEM

11. If object 1 of mass 860 kg is placed 300 m from object 2 of mass 650 kg, what force of attraction exists between the two objects?
    A. 1.24×10^{-7} N
    B. 2.48×10^{-7} N
    C. 4.14×10^{-10} N
    D. 8.28×10^{-10} N

Answer
C—When all values are correctly placed in the universal gravitation equation, the force of attraction between the two masses is determined to be 4.14×10^{-10} N.

$$F = \frac{Gm_1 m_2}{r^2}$$

$$F = \frac{(6.67 \times 10^{-11} \text{ Nm}^2/\text{kg}^2)(860 \text{ kg})(650 \text{ kg})}{(300 \text{ m})^2}$$

$$F = \frac{0.0000372853 \text{ Nm}^2}{90,000 \text{ m}^2}$$

$$F = 4.14 \times 10^{-10} \text{ N}$$

Waves and Sound

To review waves, it is helpful to take a look at the vocabulary associated with waves in Box 8-2 and the illustration in Figure 8-3.

The frequency of the wave and the period of the wave are inversely related and expressed mathematically as follows, where f = the frequency and T = the period.

$$f = \frac{1}{T}$$

and

$$T = \frac{1}{f}$$

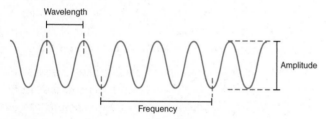

Box 8-2 Wave Vocabulary

Crest: High point of a wave.
Trough: Low point of a wave.
Amplitude: Maximum displacement from equilibrium.
Wavelength: Distance between successive identical parts of a wave.
Frequency: Vibrations or oscillations per unit of time (number of waves per unit time). Frequency is expressed in vibrations per second and is measured in hertz (s^{-1}).

FIGURE 8-3 Components of a wave. (From Johnston JN, Fauber TL: *Essentials of radiographic physics and imaging*, St. Louis, 2012, Elsevier Mosby.)

Waves are produced by objects that vibrate or show simple harmonic motion. A wave is a disturbance or pulse that travels through a medium or space. Waves are carriers of energy that travel in the form of light, sound, microwaves, ultraviolet light, x-rays, gamma rays, television, radio, and so on. There are two types of waves, mechanical and electromagnetic.

Mechanical Waves

Each type of mechanical wave is associated with some material or substance called the *medium* for that type. As the wave travels through the medium, the particles that make up the medium undergo displacements of various kinds, depending on the nature of the wave. Examples of these would be sound, water, and seismic.

Electromagnetic Waves

Electromagnetic waves do not require a medium for transmission. These waves are produced by electricity and magnetism and make up the electromagnetic spectrum. They are pure energy and travel as electric and magnetic disturbances in space (Figure 8-4). These waves all travel at the speed of light (3×10^8 m/sec). The components of the electromagnetic spectrum are radiowaves, microwaves, infrared light, visible light, ultraviolet light, x-rays, and gamma rays.

Classification of Waves

Waves are classified by the way they displace matter or how they cause matter to vibrate. The wave is either transverse or longitudinal in nature. Transverse waves are waves that cause the particles of the medium to vibrate perpendicular

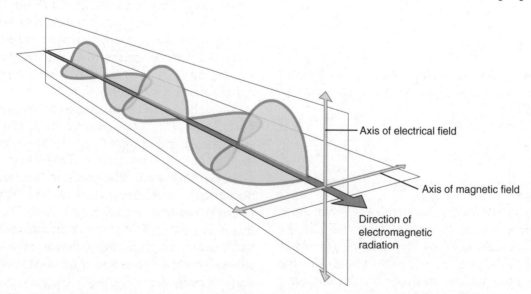

FIGURE 8-4 Electromagnetic radiation is an electric and magnetic disturbance in space. (From Johnston JN, Fauber TL: *Essentials of radiographic physics and imaging*, St. Louis, 2012, Elsevier Mosby.)

to the direction the wave travels. Longitudinal or compressional waves are waves that cause the particles of the medium to vibrate parallel to the direction of the wave. With both longitudinal and transverse waves, the particles of the medium vibrate but *do not* travel with the wave. Longitudinal waves require a medium to be transmitted. The speed at which a wave travels through a medium is determined by the frequency and the wavelength of the wave. This relationship is expressed mathematically as follows, where f = frequency and λ = the wavelength.

$$\text{Speed} = f\lambda$$

The amplitude of a wave is proportional to the potential energy content of the wave. Therefore the higher the wave, the greater the stored energy it is carrying. The higher the frequency, the more kinetic energy the wave possesses because speed $(v) = f\lambda$ and $KE = \frac{1}{2}mv^2$.

When a string is plucked, a wave will reflect back and forth from one end of the string to the other, creating nodes and antinodes. This is called a *standing wave* because it appears to stand still. Nodes are points along the standing wave that remain stationary. Antinodes are points of maximum energy where the largest amplitude occurs along the standing wave. The frequency at which the string vibrates depends on the number of antinodes, the wave speed, and the length of the vibrating string. Mathematically this relationship is expressed as follows:

$$\text{Frequency} = \frac{(\text{Number of antinodes})(\text{Wave speed})}{2(\text{Length})} = \frac{nv}{2L}$$

SAMPLE PROBLEM

12. A wave in a string travels at 24 m/sec and has a wavelength of 0.90 m. What is the frequency?
    A. 2.67 Hz
    B. 26.67 Hz
    C. 1.33 Hz
    D. 13.33 Hz

   Answer

   B—To determine the frequency of a wave given the speed and wavelength, simply divide the speed of the wave by the wavelength. After insertion of the appropriate values in the following equation, the frequency of the wave is determined to be 26.67 Hz.

$$\text{speed} = f\lambda$$

Convert the equation to solve for frequency (*f*).

$$f = \frac{\text{speed}}{\lambda}$$

$$f = \frac{24 \text{ m/sec}}{0.9 \text{ m}}$$

$$f = 26.67 \text{ Hz}$$

HESI Hint

Medical imaging, whether radiography, magnetic resonance imaging (MRI), or ultrasound, deals with electromagnetic waves/energies. An understanding of their nature and physical attributes is essential to competent practice as a medical imaging professional.

Light

Light is an electromagnetic wave that travels at 3.0×10^8 m/sec. Light needs no medium through which to travel and is a result of electric and magnetic interactions. Light exhibits properties of both a wave and a particle. When light interacts with a medium, it does so at the atomic level. The light energy is absorbed by the electrons of the atoms causing them to vibrate. This excess energy may be absorbed by the medium and converted to heat. It may also be reflected or it may be transmitted (pass through with some refraction or bending). For example, when light traveling through air reaches a mirror the mirror constitutes a new boundary, a transition from one medium (air) to another (glass mirror). At this boundary, some of the light energy will be reflected and some will be transmitted into this new medium. We are mainly interested in two properties of light: reflection and refraction.

Reflection is the bouncing back of a wave from a barrier or from a boundary between two media as depicted in Figure 8-5. There are a few terms important to the discussion of reflection. Incident wave is the wave that strikes the barrier (or boundary). Reflected wave is the wave that bounces off and leaves the barrier. The normal line is a reference line that is drawn perpendicular to a barrier. The angle of incidence is the angle between the normal line and the incident wave. The angle of reflection is the angle between the normal line and the reflected wave. Applying the mirror example to Figure 8-5, the mirror would be the

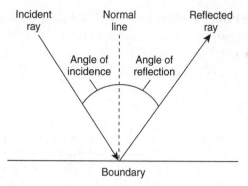

FIGURE 8-5 Reflection is a wave bouncing back from a barrier or from a boundary between two media.

boundary, the incident ray would be the light traveling to the mirror, and the reflected ray is the light traveling way from the mirror. The law of reflection states that when a wave disturbance is reflected at a boundary of a transmitting medium, the angle of incidence must equal the angle of reflection.

HESI Hint

X-rays and gamma rays also exhibit properties of both a wave and a particle referred to as *wave/particle duality*. Understanding this property aids in understanding how these radiant energies interact with matter.

Refraction is the bending of a wave as it passes at an angle from one medium into another if the speed of propagation differs. That is, refraction is caused by the change in speed of a wave as it transitions from one medium to the next. Figure 8-6 depicts a light ray as it passes from air into a container of water. Different media

have different speeds of propagation, so light travels at different speeds through different media. Which way light will refract relative to normal depends on whether the wave is transitioning to a faster or slower medium. As waves move from one medium into an optically denser medium (from a faster medium to a slower medium), the wave bends toward the normal. As waves move from a medium into an optically less dense medium (from a slower medium to a faster medium), the wave bends away from the normal.

The mathematic relationship for this behavior is called *Snell's law*, which is expressed mathematically as follows, where n = the index of refraction and θ = the angle of refraction.

$$n_1 \sin\theta_1 = n_2 \sin\theta_2$$

The index of refraction is a ratio of the speed of light in a vacuum to the speed of light in a given material. This mathematic relationship is expressed as follows, where c = the speed of light in a vacuum (3×10^8 m/sec) and v_s = the speed of light in a given substance.

$$n = \frac{c}{v_s}$$

SAMPLE PROBLEM

13. If the index of refraction for quartz is 1.46, what is the speed of light in quartz?
    A. 2.05×10^8 m/sec
    B. 4.38×10^8 m/sec
    C. 1.25×10^8 m/sec
    D. 0.489×10^8 m/sec

Answer
A—To determine the speed of light in quartz, divide the speed of light by index of refraction for quartz. Through use of the following equation, the speed of light in quartz is determined to be 2.05×10^8 m/sec.

$$n = \frac{c}{v_s}$$

Convert the equation to solve for speed of light in a substance (v_s).

$$v_s = \frac{3 \times 10^8 \text{ m/sec}}{1.46}$$

$$v_s = 2.05 \times 10^8 \text{ m/sec}$$

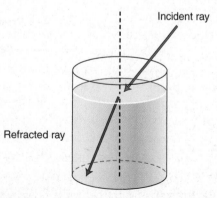

FIGURE 8-6 Light ray refracted in a container of water.

Optics

The previous discussion of reflection assumed a plane mirror. While still obeying the law of reflection, the shape of the mirror, specifically spherical mirrors (i.e., convex or concave), changes the direction of reflection. Concave mirrors have positive focal lengths, whereas convex mirrors have negative focal lengths. Concave mirrors form a variety of image shapes, sizes, and orientations, depending on the focal length of the mirror and where the object is placed. Figure 8-7 depicts a concave mirror with the focal point (*f*) and curvature (*C*). With the object beyond the center of curvature (*C*), we have an image that is smaller than the object and inverted in orientation. If we place the object at *C*, the resulting image is the same size as the object and inverted in orientation. If the object is between *C* and the focal point (*f*), the image is larger than the object and inverted in orientation. If the object is at *f*, there is no image formed. If the object is between *f* and the mirror, the image is upright and larger in size and virtual. Convex mirrors can form only images that are smaller and upright. Real images are always inverted, and virtual images are always upright.

Lenses form images by refraction. There are two basic types of lenses: convex (converging) and concave (diverging). Convex lenses always have positive focal lengths, and concave lenses always have negative focal lengths. Convex lenses can form a variety of image shapes, sizes, and orientations, depending on the focal length of the lens and the object's position. When an object is placed at a position greater than *2f*, the image is reduced, inverted, and on the opposite side of the lens. The placement of an object at *2f* results in an image that is the same size as the object, inverted, and on the opposite side of the lens. The placement of an object between *2f* and *f* results in an image that is larger than the object, inverted, and on the opposite side of the lens. When the object is placed at *f*, no image is formed.

If the object is between *f* and the lens, the image is upright, larger, and on the same side of the lens. A concave lens can form only an image that is upright and smaller than the object.

Atomic Structure

Many discussions of physical principles are aided by an understanding of basic atomic structure. The atom is composed of three fundamental particles: protons, neutrons, and electrons (Figure 8-8). Protons are one part of the nucleus of the atom and carry one unit of positive electric charge. Neutrons are the other principal part of the nucleus and are electrically neutral. Electrons orbit the nucleus in specific energy levels and carry one unit of negative electric charge. The energy levels or shells in which the electrons orbit are lettered beginning with "k" (i.e., k, l, m, n, o etc.). The closer the electron shell the stronger the **binding energy** (how tightly the electron is bound to the nucleus). Each shell holds a specific number of electrons. This number may be found using the following formula, where *n* is the shell number (k = 1, l = 2, m = 3, and so on):

$$2n^2$$

When the number of positive charges (protons in the nucleus) equals the number of negative charges (electrons in orbit), the atom is said to be stable.

HESI Hint

A solid understanding of the atom and atomic structure is key to understanding x-ray production, radiation dose, image production, and many other fundamental principles of medical imaging.

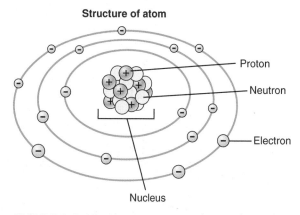

FIGURE 8-8   Basic atomic structure. (From Johnston JN, Fauber TL: *Essentials of radiographic physics and imaging*, St. Louis, 2012, Elsevier Mosby.)

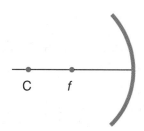

FIGURE 8-7   Concave mirror.

The Nature of Electricity

The electric property of a given material depends on the nature of its atoms. Materials whose atoms have loosely bound **valence electrons** (electrons in the outermost shell) are good conductors of electricity. Conversely, materials whose valence electrons are tightly bound are good electric insulators. Because the protons (positive charges) of an atom are tightly bound in the nucleus of the atom and not free to move about, most discussions of the flow of electricity involve negative charges (electrons).

Coulomb's Law

There are two types of basic electric charge: positive and negative. The smallest unit of positive charge rests with the proton and the smallest unit of negative charge rests with the electron. Like charges will repel each other, whereas opposite charges will attract. This force of attraction or repulsion is expressed by Coulomb's law, which states that the force of attraction or repulsion between two charged objects is directly proportional to the product of their quantities and inversely proportional to the square of the distance between them. The unit of measure for electric charge is the coulomb. The force of attraction or repulsion is determined by the mathematic relationship expressed by Coulomb's law, where k = a constant (9×10^9 N-m^2/C^2), q_1 and q_2 = the charges on objects 1 and 2 expressed in coulombs, and r = the distance between the two charged objects in meters.

$$F = \frac{k\, q_1\, q_2}{r^2}$$

SAMPLE PROBLEM

14. An object of charge 16 μC is placed 50 cm from an object of charge 30 μC. What is the magnitude of the resulting force between the two objects?
    A. 17.28 N
    B. 8.64 N
    C. 1.73×10^{13} N
    D. 8.64×10^{12} N

    Answer
    A—To solve this problem use Coulomb's law. First, convert μC to C, remembering that 1 μC is 1×10^{-6} C, and convert the distance from centimeters to meters. After insertion of the correct values into the equation, remembering to square the distance (r^2), the force between the two objects is determined to be 17.28 N.

$$F = \frac{k\, q_1\, q_2}{r^2}$$

$$F = \frac{(9 \times 10^9 \text{ N-m}^2/\text{C}^2)(16 \times 10^{-6} \text{ C})(30 \times 10^{-6} \text{ C})}{(0.5 \text{ m})^2}$$

$$F = \frac{(9 \times 10^9 \text{ N-m}^2/\text{C}^2)(16 \times 10^{-6} \text{ C})(30 \times 10^{-6} \text{ C})}{(0.5 \text{ m})^2}$$

$$F = 17.28 \text{ N}$$

Electric Fields

An electric field exists around charged objects. This field force created by the charged object is basically a change in the space that surrounds the charged object. One way to test the nature of this electric field is to use a positive test charge. If the electric field is generated by a negative charge, the test charge would experience an attractive force. If the electric field is generated by a positive charge, the test charge would experience a repulsive force. Owing to these interactions, scientists have defined the direction of an electric field to be away from a positive charge and toward a negative charge. The magnitude of an electric field is stated mathematically as follows, where E = the magnitude of the electric field, F = the force a test charge would experience, and q_o = the magnitude of the test charge.

$$E = \frac{F}{q_o}$$

Because electric fields are vector quantities, they should be treated as such. The direction of an electric field is defined as the direction a positive test charge would be moved when placed in the electric field.

SAMPLE PROBLEM

15. An electric field of magnitude 280,000 N/C points due east at a certain spot. What are the magnitude and direction of the force that acts on a charge of −10 μC?
    A. 2.8 N to the west
    B. 2.8 N to the east
    C. 28 N to the west
    D. 28 N to the east

Answer

A—To determine the magnitude of the force (F) acting on the charge, multiply the magnitude of the electric field (E) by the magnitude of the test charge (q_o). Because the charge is negative, it acts opposite to the direction of the electric field. After insertion of the appropriate values in the electric field equation, the magnitude of the charge is determined to be 2.8 N to the west.

$$E = \frac{F}{q_o}$$

Convert the equation to solve for the force (F) the test charge will experience:

$$
\begin{aligned}
F &= Eq_o \\
F &= (280,000 \text{ N/C}) \, (-10 \, \mu C) \\
&\text{Remember that 1 } \mu C \text{ is } 1 \times 10^{-6} \text{ C.} \\
F &= (280,000 \text{ N/C}) \, (-10 \, \mu C) \\
F &= (280,000 \text{ N/C}) \, (-0.00001 \text{ C}) \\
F &= -2.8 \text{ N}
\end{aligned}
$$

The negative sign in the answer indicates the direction of the force relative to the electric field.

$$F = 2.8 \text{ N to the west}$$

Nature and Properties of Circuits

An electric circuit is basically a series of electronic devices or circuit elements connected by a conductive wire that allows electric charges to continuously flow. For there to be continuous flow, there must be a conductive pathway from the positive terminal to the negative terminal and there must be a potential difference between the terminals. The flow of current is determined by the voltage available and the resistance of the circuit. The mathematic relationship between voltage, current, and resistance is known as *Ohm's law*, which states that the potential difference (voltage) in a circuit or any part of that circuit is equal to the current (amperes) multiplied by the resistance (ohms). Ohm's law is expressed as follows, where V = potential difference in voltage expressed in volts, I = current expressed in amperes, and R = resistance expressed in ohms.

$$V = IR$$

Voltage is an expression of the potential difference between two points and is measured in volts. A volt is the work (in joules) that may be done per unit of charge. Current is measured in amperes, which is defined as one coulomb of electricity flowing by a given point in one second. Resistance is measured in ohms and is that property of a circuit element that impedes the flow of electricity. One ohm is equal to the resistance between two points necessary to allow a current of one ampere when one volt is applied.

There are two types of basic circuits: series circuits and parallel circuits. A series circuit has only one pathway through which current can flow, so current is the same through all resistors. A parallel circuit has several pathways through which current can flow, but all resistors are connected directly to the same battery, so the voltage supplied for each resistor is the same. To determine the total resistance of a series circuit, you would add the individual resistors. To determine the total resistance of a parallel circuit, you would add the reciprocal of the individual resistors and then take the reciprocal of that value. Once the total resistance is determined and the type of circuit used is known, the current flowing through each resistor can be determined.

SAMPLE PROBLEM

16. A circuit consists of a 10-ohm resistor, a 15-ohm resistor, and a 25-ohm resistor. The resistors are placed in series and then wired to a 100-V power supply. Determine the current flowing in the circuit.
    A. 0.5 amp
    B. 2.0 amp
    C. 10.0 amp
    D. 4.0 amp

Answer

B—Before the current flowing through the circuit is determined, the total resistance must be calculated. Because the resistors are placed in a series, the total resistance is determined by adding the individual values of the individual resistors.

$$
\begin{aligned}
\text{Total Resistance}_{(\text{in a series})} &= R_1 + R_2 + R_3 \\
\text{Total Resistance}_{(\text{in a series})} &= 10 \text{ ohm} + 15 \text{ ohm} + \\
&\quad 25 \text{ ohm} \\
\text{Total Resistance}_{(\text{in a series})} &= 50 \text{ ohm}
\end{aligned}
$$

To determine the current in the circuit, use the Ohm's law equation. After insertion of the appropriate values into the equation, the

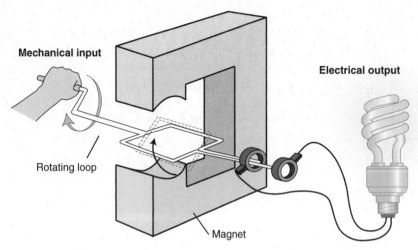

Mechanical input

Electrical output

Rotating loop

Magnet

FIGURE 8-9   A conductor rotated in a magnetic field will generate electricity. (From Johnston JN, Fauber TL: *Essentials of radiographic physics and imaging*, St. Louis, 2012, Elsevier Mosby.)

current flowing in the circuit is determined to be 2.0 amp.

$$V = IR$$

Convert the equation to solve for current (*I*).

$$I = \frac{100 \text{ Volts}}{50 \text{ ohms}}$$

$$I = 2.0 \text{ amps}$$

Magnetism and Electricity

Magnetism is that property of a material that will attract iron, cobalt, or nickel. Magnetic fields exist as lines of force in space known as *flux*. These flux lines create elliptical loops in space that extend from the north pole externally to the south pole of the magnet. As with electric charges, like magnetic poles repel each other and opposite magnetic poles attract. Additionally, the force of attraction or repulsion between two magnetic fields varies directly as the strength of the magnetic poles and inversely as the square of the

distance between them. The strength of a magnetic field is measured in Teslas.

Electricity and magnetism are two parts of the same basic force known as electromagnetism. That is, any flow of electricity, whether in space or in a conductor, will create around it an associated magnetic field. Likewise, any moving magnetic field will create an electric current. This induction of an electric current is known as *electromagnetic induction*. When a conductor is passed back and forth in a magnetic field or the flux from a moving magnetic field passes through a conductor, an electric current will be induced to flow in that conductor. Figure 8-9 demonstrates a conductor being rotated in a magnetic field that induces current in the loop to power the light bulb.

HESI Hint

Magnetism and electricity are fundamental to x-ray production. There is no magical process involved in the production of x-rays by medical imaging equipment. It is simply the manipulation of electricity.

MATHEMATICS PRACTICE TEST

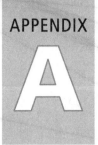

1. Evaluate

   $ab^2 - ac$ if $a = 3, b = -4,$ and $c = -5$

2. Evaluate

   $3x^2 - 2x + 7$ if $x = -3$.

3. Solve for x:

   $-7x + 9 = -47$

4. Solve for t:

   $50 = -3t - 7$

5. A newborn weighs 8 pounds 5 ounces. There are 453.59 grams per pound. What is the infant's weight in grams?
   A. 2268 grams
   B. 3629 grams
   C. 3770 grams
   D. 3856 grams

6. What temperature in Fahrenheit is 50° Celsius? (Enter numeric value only. If rounding is necessary, round to the nearest whole number.) _____

7. A nurse works in a military hospital from 1300 to 2000. What time of day does this nurse work?
   A. Early morning to early afternoon
   B. Lunch time to midnight
   C. Early afternoon to bedtime
   D. Midnight to sunrise

8. A nurse is reviewing the daily intake and output (I&O) of a patient consuming a clear diet. The urinary drainage bag denotes a total of 1,000 mL for the past 24 hours. The total intake is:
   2 8-oz cups of coffee
   1 16-oz serving of clear soup
   1 pint of water consumed throughout the day
   How much is the deficit in milliliters? (Enter numeric value only. If rounding is necessary, round to the nearest whole number.)
   _____

9. A woman received a bottle of perfume as a present. The bottle contains ½ oz of perfume. How many milliliters is this? (Enter numeric value only. If rounding is necessary, round to the nearest whole number.)

   _____

10. The metric system of measurement was developed in France during Napoleon's reign. It is based on what multiplication factor?
    A. The length of Napoleon's forearm
    B. 2
    C. 10
    D. Atomic weight of helium

11. How many meters are in a kilometer? (Enter numeric value only.) _____

12. How many grams are in a kilogram? (Enter numeric value only.) _____

13. To convert pounds to kilograms, what factor is used?
    A. 2.2
    B. 0.334
    C. 10
    D. 22

14. A teacher's aide is preparing a snack for the class. In order to prepare the powdered drink, the aide must convert the directions from metric. The directions say, "Dilute contents of package in 2 liters of water." The aide has a measuring device marked in ounces. How many ounces of water should be used? (Enter numeric value only. If rounding is required, round to the nearest tenth.) _____

15. How many milliliters are in 1 liter?
    A. 30
    B. 10
    C. 100
    D. 1,000

16. There are 2.54 cm in an inch. How many centimeters are in 1 foot? (Enter numeric value only. If rounding is necessary, round to the nearest whole number.) _____

17. A seamstress is measuring a model for a new dress. The tape measure is marked in centimeters. The seamstress needs to convert that measurement into inches. If the model's waist measurement is 65.4 cm, what is the conversion in inches?
    A. 25.74 inches
    B. 166.12 inches
    C. 32.50 inches
    D. 17 inches

18. How many centimeters in a millimeter?
    A. $\frac{1}{10}$
    B. 1
    C. 10
    D. 100

19. How many centimeters in a meter?
    A. $\frac{1}{100}$
    B. 10
    C. 100
    D. 1,000

20. A news website allows subscribers to download news articles in different languages. The average number of downloads per day for some of the languages are as follows:
    English: 5 articles, 150 downloads
    French: 2 articles, 50 downloads
    Chinese: 1 article, 75 downloads
    Japanese: 3 articles, 25 downloads
    How many articles are downloaded each day?

21. A hospital day staff consists of 25 registered nurses, 75 unlicensed assistants, five phlebologists, six receptionists and office staff, and 45 physicians. One summer day the staff was at only 68% strength. How many people were working that day? (Enter numeric value only. If rounding is necessary, round to the nearest whole number.) _____

22. A farmer raises chickens for eggs and meat. Any chicken that does not lay at least one egg a week is moved to the slaughterhouse. The farmer has 765 chickens that can lay one egg each day. Each day 80% of the chickens lay eggs. How many eggs does the farmer collect each day? (Enter numeric value only. If rounding is necessary, round to the nearest whole number.) _____

23. Over the past week, 34 baby boys were born at the hospital. This was 54% of all babies born. How many girls were born over the past week? (Enter numeric value only. If rounding is necessary, round to the nearest whole number.) _____

24. The doctor tells the patient to cut back on coffee. The patient usually has four 8-oz cups of coffee per day. If the doctor told him to cut back by 25%, how many ounces of coffee can the patient have each day? (Enter numeric value only. If rounding is necessary, round to the whole number.) _____

25. Ratio and proportion: 0.8:10 :: x:100
    A. x = 0.8
    B. x = 8
    C. x = 80
    D. x = 800

26. Add: 9.98 + 0.065 =
    A. 10.63
    B. 10.045
    C. 1.0063
    D. 998.065

27. Add: 6 + 12.55 + 5.022 =
    A. 18.55
    B. 23.572
    C. 30.025
    D. 16.475

28. Add: 23.5 + 7.025 =
    A. 30.525
    B. 30.5
    C. 30.025
    D. 16.475

29. Subtract: 32.21 − 4.68 =
    A. 14.59
    B. 27.53
    C. 1.459
    D. 31.742

30. Subtract: 15.7 − 9.8 =
    A. 6.1
    B. 8.96
    C. 5.9
    D. 4.30

31. Subtract: 10.012 − 0.120 =
    A. 10
    B. 9.012
    C. 10.122
    D. 9.892

32. Multiply: (7.2)(0.34) =
    A. 14.12
    B. 0.234
    C. 7.64
    D. 2.448

33. Multiply: (99)(0.56) =
    A. 99.30
    B. 99.56
    C. 55.44
    D. 199.54

34. Multiply: (88)(7.08) =
    A. 862.5
    B. 88.040

C. 64.252
D. 623.04

35. Multiply: 375 × 2.3 =
    A. 862.5
    B. 750
    C. 225.75
    D. 1125

36. How many ounces are in 2 quarts?
    A. 8 ounces
    B. 16 ounces
    C. 32 ounces
    D. 64 ounces

37. A shopper spends $75.64 at one store and $22.43 at the next store. The shopper started out with $100.00. How much money does the shopper have left?
    A. $1.93
    B. $5.00
    C. $0.72
    D. $20.13

38. A worker is filling out his timesheet. He worked 8 hours on Monday, 7 hours and 30 minutes on Tuesday, 8¾ hours on Wednesday, 4 hours on Thursday, and 8¼ hours on Friday. If he earns $14.35 per hour, what will be his gross pay for this week? (Enter numeric value only. Round your answer to the nearest penny.)

    _____

39. An accountant counts his money and finds that out of 35 bills, 20% are $1 bills, 43% are $5 bills, 6% are $10 bills, and 31% are $20 bills. How many $5 bills does the accountant have? (Enter numeric value only. If rounding is necessary, round to the nearest whole number.) _____

40. What number in Arabic numerals is Roman numeral MCMXLIV? (Enter numeric value only.) _____

MATHEMATICS ANSWER KEY

1. 63
2. 40
3. x = 8
4. t = −19
5. C
6. 122° F
7. C
8. 440
9. 15
10. C
11. 1,000
12. 1,000
13. A
14. 66.7
15. D
16. 30.48
17. A
18. A
19. C
20. 1000

21. 106
22. 612
23. 29
24. 24
25. B
26. B
27. B
28. A
29. B
30. C
31. D
32. D
33. C
34. D
35. A
36. D
37. A
38. 523.78
39. 15
40. 1,944

READING COMPREHENSION PRACTICE TEST

 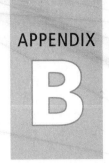

Blood Pressure

Lub-dub! Lub-dub! Lub-dub! This sound is made by the rapid contracting and extending of the chamber doors on the inside of the heart. This ventricular contracting injects roughly 70 mL of blood into a vascular system with a given volume at differing pressure.

Blood pressure refers to the pressure in the arterial system; and it is typically taken in the brachial artery of the arm because the pressure at different places along the circulatory route is different. Blood pressure is simply the force that the blood exerts in all directions within any given area and is the basis for the movement of blood from the heart, through the body, and back to the heart. This pressure is commonly expressed as a ratio of the systolic pressure over the diastolic pressure.

The systolic pressure or "high peak" pressure takes place within the arterial system as ventricles contract and force blood into the arteries. The diastolic pressure or "low peak" pressure takes place within this arterial system just before the next ventricular contraction.

An increase in blood pressure can occur if the arterial walls lose some of their elasticity with age or disease.

1. What is the main idea of the passage?
    A. Blood pressure overall measures the elasticity of the arteries near the heart as they stretch to accommodate expelled blood.
    B. Blood pressure within the arterial system takes into account that pressure is different at varying locations.
    C. Blood pressure is simply the force that the blood exerts in all directions within any given area, measured as a ratio.
    D. Blood pressure represents the pulse difference between ventricular contractions.

2. Which statement is not a detail from the passage?
    A. The ventricular contraction asserts capillary pressure that is about 70 mm Hg.
    B. The pressures at different places in the circulatory system are different.
    C. Increase in blood pressure can occur if arterial walls lose some of their elasticity.
    D. Blood pressure is expressed as a ratio of systolic over diastolic pressure.

3. What is the meaning of the word *elasticity* in the last paragraph?
    A. Something that is able to resist and be flexible
    B. Something that is like plastic
    C. Something that is dynamic and electrifying
    D. Something that is silly

4. What is the author's primary purpose in writing this essay?
    A. To entertain the reader with information about the blood system
    B. To analyze how blood pressure can affect an individual's health
    C. To inform the reader how blood pressure is measured
    D. To persuade the reader of the importance of accurate blood pressure procedures

5. Which of the following is not a fact stated in the passage?
   A. Ventricular contracting injects roughly 70 mL of blood into a vascular system.
   B. Blood pressure is typically taken in the brachial artery of the arm.
   C. Blood pressure is commonly expressed as a ratio of the systolic pressure over the diastolic pressure.
   D. Loss of arterial wall elasticity is always caused by disease.

6. Which is the best summary of this passage?
   A. The heart pumps roughly 70 mL of blood by rapidly contracting and extending the chamber doors of the heart. Disease and age affect the pressure of blood on arterial walls.
   B. The brachial artery of the arm is usually used to take blood pressure, although the pressure is different in different parts of the body.
   C. The measurement of the ratio of systolic pressure over the diastolic pressure is known as *blood pressure.*
   D. The force that blood exerts on arterial walls is known as *blood pressure* and is measured as a ratio of the systolic pressure or "high peak" over the diastolic pressure or "low peak."

Blood Pressure Regulators

The body is composed of systems that have evolved and diversified in order to maintain the natural functions and processes they regulate. One such system that has these regulators is the body's cardiovascular system. The body's pump, which regulates the flow of vitally needed oxygen to all cells of the body, as well as the discard of carbon dioxide and other waste products, is the heart.

Because blood pressure varies at different points within the body, differing components are needed to keep the body's blood pressure regulated. Three of the basic components are baroreceptors, chemoreceptors, and the kidneys.

Baroreceptors are stretch receptors composed of fine branching nerve endings and are contained along the walls of the arteries near the heart and in other areas of the body as well. Impulses are related to this stretching along the arterial walls, which causes these baroreceptors to send out even more impulses to the heart, arteries, and veins, causing the blood pressure to go either up or down.

Chemoreceptors are located along the walls of the arteries and monitor changes in oxygen level, carbon dioxide, and pH. Just think! A fall in oxygen causes receptors to send impulses to raise the blood pressure.

The kidneys play a role in regulating blood pressure by absorbing salts and water and removing wastes. Hormones secreted by the adrenal cortex cause the kidney to keep or let go of any salt and water. This has an influence on blood volume and consequently on blood pressure.

7. What is the main idea of the passage?
   A. Blood pressure can be treated only by monitoring baroreceptors.
   B. Blood pressure can be treated only by monitoring chemoreceptors.
   C. Blood pressure can be treated only by monitoring the kidneys.
   D. Blood pressure can be regulated through baroreceptors, chemoreceptors, and the kidneys.

8. Which statement is not a detail from the passage?
   A. Baroreceptors are rigid and static nerve endings that are contained along the arterial walls and send out messages along the nerve pathway.
   B. Chemoreceptors are located along the walls of the arteries and monitor changes in oxygen level.
   C. The kidneys play a role in regulating blood pressure by absorbing salts and water.
   D. The heart is the body's pump, which regulates the flow of vitally needed oxygen to cells of the body.

9. What is the meaning of the word *evolved* in the first paragraph?
   A. To spread
   B. To gradually develop
   C. To revolve
   D. To shift

10. What is the writer's primary purpose in writing this essay?
    A. To inform the reader about the dangers of high blood pressure
    B. To inform the reader how high blood pressure leads to a higher risk of heart attack
    C. To inform the reader how the cardiovascular system regulates blood pressure
    D. To persuade the reader that controlling one's blood pressure is important

11. What is the best summary of this passage?
    A. The body's pump, the heart, regulates the flow of oxygen to all cells of the body and discards waste products that include carbon dioxide. The kidneys help in this process by absorbing salts and water.
    B. There are several systems to maintain the natural functions and processes of the body. One system is the cardiovascular system, which regulates blood pressure through baroreceptors, chemoreceptors, and the kidneys.
    C. Baroreceptors help regulate blood pressure and are found along the wall of the arteries. Baroreceptors send out impulses to the heart, arteries, and veins, resulting in the lowering or raising of blood pressure.
    D. Chemoreceptors monitor changes in oxygen level that affect blood pressure.

12. What is a major difference in the way baroreceptors and chemoreceptors work from the way the kidneys work?
    A. Baroreceptors and chemoreceptors both work within the wall of the arteries sending out impulses to raise or lower blood pressure, whereas the kidneys help control blood volume.
    B. Baroreceptors and chemoreceptors both work to help maintain blood volume, whereas the kidneys take care of salts, water, and waste removal.
    C. Baroreceptors and chemoreceptors must work together to control blood pressure, whereas the kidneys work with the adrenal cortex.
    D. Baroreceptors and chemoreceptors are both located near the adrenal cortex, whereas the kidneys are located near the heart.

Doppler Effect

Have you ever wondered why the whistle of a traveling, distant locomotive predicts its approach several yards before anyone actually sees it? Or why an oncoming ambulance's screaming siren is heard momentarily several feet before the ambulance comes into full view, before it passes you, and why its siren is still heard faintly well after the ambulance is out of sight?

What you are witnessing is a scientific phenomenon known as the *Doppler effect*. What takes place is truly remarkable. In both of these instances, when the train or ambulance moves toward the sound waves in front of it, the sound waves are pulled closer together and have a higher frequency. In either instance, the listener positioned in front of the moving object hears a higher pitch. The ambulance and locomotive are progressively moving away from the sound waves behind them, causing the waves to be farther apart and to have a lower frequency. These fast-approaching modes of transportation distance themselves past the listener, who hears a lower pitch.

13. Which statement is not listed as a detail in the passage?
    A. The oncoming sound waves have a higher pitch because of high frequency and closeness of waves.
    B. The oncoming sound waves have a higher pitch because of low frequency and closeness of waves.
    C. The whistling sound of the locomotive as it approaches and passes can be explained by the Doppler effect.
    D. The high-pitched sound of the ambulance as it approaches and passes can be explained by the Doppler effect.

14. What is the main idea of the passage?
    A. Trains and ambulances make distinctly loud noises.
    B. Low-frequency waves make high-pitched sounds.
    C. High-frequency waves make low-pitched sounds.
    D. The Doppler effect explains the rationale for why sound is heard initially more strongly and then faintly after a moving object has passed.

15. What is the meaning of the word *phenomenon* in the second paragraph?
    A. Something that is lifeless to the senses
    B. Something that is nonchalant
    C. Something that is significant but unusual
    D. Something that is chemical in origin

16. What is the author's primary purpose in writing this essay?
    A. To entertain the reader with information about trains and ambulances
    B. To inform the reader about avoiding accidents, which involve trains and ambulances
    C. To inform the reader about how movement affects sound
    D. To analyze the difference between train and ambulance sounds

17. Which sound waves have a higher pitch?
    A. Those waves that are closer together
    B. Those waves that are farther apart
    C. Those waves that travel a long distance
    D. Those waves that travel a short distance

18. Which sound waves have a lower pitch?
    A. Those waves that are closer together
    B. Those waves that are farther apart
    C. Those waves that travel a long distance
    D. Those waves that travel a short distance

Electrocardiogram

Beep!...Beep!...Beep! is the audible rhythmic sound made as the strength of the heart muscle is measured. The signal cadence has a characteristic record that varies in every individual. This record is called an *electrocardiogram,* or ECG.

In the body, an array of systemic neural responses constantly occur, emitting electric currents. The electric currents can be detected on the surface of the body, and if a person is hooked to an amplifier, these impulses are recorded by an electrocardiograph.

Most of the information obtained is about the heart because the heart sends out electric currents in waves. This "wave of excitation" spreads through the heart wall and is accompanied by electric changes. The wave takes place in three distinct steps.

Initially, the "wave of excitation" accompanied by an electric change lasts for approximately 1 to 2 seconds after the contraction of the cardiac muscle. The electric impulses are discharged rhythmically from the sinoatrial (SA) node, the pacemaker of the heart. This spread of excitation over the muscle of the atrium indicates that the atrium has contracted.

Next, the peak of the ECG reading is due to the atrioventricular (AV) node, causing the ventricle to become excited.

Finally, the ventricles relax, and any changes in the wave indicate to trained medical staff any abnormalities within the heart.

19. What is the author's primary purpose in writing the essay?
    A. To persuade the reader to have an ECG
    B. To entertain the reader with a heart-warming story
    C. To inform the reader how an electrocardiograph reads the electric currents emitted by the heart
    D. To analyze the difference in the SA node and the AV node

20. Which statement is not listed as a detail within the passage?
    A. Changes in the ECG are typically used for diagnosis of abnormal cardiac rhythm.
    B. The signal has a characteristic record called the *electrocardiogram.*
    C. The "wave of excitation" starts at the SA node.
    D. The "wave of excitation" spreads through the heart wall and is accompanied by electric changes.

21. What is the meaning of the word *emitting* as it is used in the second paragraph?
    A. Repelling
    B. Releasing
    C. Closing
    D. Charging

22. What is the main idea of the passage?
    A. Electric currents within the body are due to electrostatic charges set off by the heart.
    B. The ECG systematically and quickly measures the stages at which the "wave of excitation" occurs within the heart and records them.

C. The "wave of excitation" is detected on the surface of the body and is used to measure the atrial excitation of the heart.

D. The electric currents within the body are in direct relation to the "wave of excitation" measured by the ECG.

23. What is the best summary of the passage?
A. Electric currents within the body are due to electrostatic charges set off by the heart. Medical staff are trained to recognize any abnormalities within the heart.
B. Every individual has unique electric currents on the surface of the body. The ECG measures and records these electric currents.
C. The ECG systematically and rather quickly measures the stages at which the "wave of excitation" occurs within the heart and records them. This wave has three distinct steps that spread from the SA node to the AV node.
D. The ECG measures the electric currents within the body. These currents are detected on the surface of the body when the body is connected to an amplifier.

24. What are the three steps of the "wave of excitation"?
A. The discharge from the SA node, the peak ECG, and the excitement of the ventricle.
B. The excitement of the ventricle, the relaxing of the ventricle, and the systemic neural response.
C. The contraction of the atrium, the relaxation of the atrium, and the contraction of the ventricle.
D. The excitation of the atrium, the excitement of the ventricle, and the relaxing of the ventricle.

The Water Cycle

Water is needed to sustain practically all life functions on planet Earth. A single drop of this compound is composed of an oxygen atom that shares its electrons with each of the two hydrogen atoms.

The cycle starts when precipitation, such as rain, snow, sleet, or hail, descends from the sky onto the ground. Water that is not absorbed immediately from the precipitation is known as *runoff*. The runoff flows across the land and collects in groundwater reservoirs, rivers, streams, and oceans.

Evaporation takes place when liquid water changes into water vapor, which is a gas. Water vapor returns to the air from surface water and plants.

Ultimately, condensation happens when this water vapor cools and changes back into droplets of liquid. In fact, the puffy, cotton clouds that we observe are formed by condensation. When the clouds become heavily laden with liquid droplets, precipitation ensues.

25. What is the meaning of the word *composed* in the first paragraph?
A. To consist of
B. To be uniquely discovered
C. To be set apart
D. To be surprised

26. What is the main idea of this passage?
A. Water is formed from the joining of two hydrogen atoms to one atom of oxygen.
B. Water is a versatile and important universal solvent.
C. The different components of the water cycle are precipitation, evaporation, and condensation.
D. Rain is a trivial part of the life cycle.

27. Which statement is not a detail from the passage?
A. A single drop of water is made of a couple of hydrogen atoms and oxygen atoms.
B. Evaporation takes place when liquid water changes into water vapor.
C. Water that is not absorbed is called *runoff*.
D. Condensation fails to happen when water vapor cools and changes back into droplets of liquid.

28. What was the author's primary purpose for writing this essay?
A. To persuade the reader to conserve water
B. To persuade the reader that runoff is not the best way to collect water
C. To analyze different types of runoff
D. To inform the reader about the stages of the water cycle

29. What can the reader conclude from this passage about ponds and lakes?
    A. They are examples of groundwater reservoirs.
    B. They are not important in the collection of runoff.
    C. They do not play a role in water collection.
    D. They consist of only water collected through precipitation.

30. Knowing that the cooling of water vapor results in condensation, one could conclude that _____ is/are a factor in the evaporation process.

    A. Humidity
    B. Heat
    C. Electrons
    D. Runoff

READING COMPREHENSION PRACTICE TEST ANSWER KEY

1. C	16. C
2. A	17. A
3. A	18. B
4. C	19. C
5. D	20. A
6. D	21. B
7. D	22. B
8. A	23. C
9. B	24. D
10. C	25. A
11. B	26. C
12. A	27. D
13. B	28. D
14. D	29. A
15. C	30. B

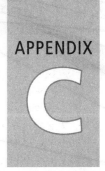
VOCABULARY PRACTICE TEST

1. Select the meaning of the underlined word in the sentence.
   The nurse called the doctor when the patient's condition began to <u>deteriorate</u>.
   A. grow
   B. improve
   C. worsen
   D. clarify

2. Select the meaning of the underlined word in the sentence.
   The patient was diagnosed with a psychiatric <u>disorder</u>.
   A. rule
   B. system
   C. organization
   D. illness

3. Select the word that means "brief, to the point."
   The teacher's instructions were concise, so the student was able to complete the project in a reasonable period of time.
   A. period
   B. concise
   C. complete
   D. reasonable

4. What word meaning "once a year" fits best in the sentence?
   The _____ family reunion picnic was held at the Jones farm instead of the county park.
   A. regular
   B. annual
   C. biennial
   D. holiday

5. Docile is best defined as being _____.
   A. defiant
   B. disobedient
   C. firm
   D. compliant

6. Select the meaning of the underlined word in the sentence.
   Because the patient had an <u>occluded</u> artery, the physician decided to perform cardiovascular surgery.
   A. Obstructed
   B. Open
   C. Broken
   D. Cloudy

7. Select the word that means "an undesired problem that is the result of some other event."
   The complication of the surgery caused the patient to remain in the hospital to have an additional complement of testing procedures implemented.
   A. Complication
   B. Complement
   C. Procedures
   D. Implemented

8. Select the meaning of the underlined word in the sentence.
   The dog developed <u>bilateral</u> weakness in its hindquarters, so the veterinarian created a wheeled cart to help the dog walk.
   A. Present on two sides
   B. Available for exercise
   C. Affecting the left side
   D. Affecting the right side

9. Select the correct definition of the underlined word.
   The doctor's <u>prognosis</u> gave the patient and his family reason to feel optimistic about the surgery.
   A. Instructions
   B. Estimate
   C. Behavior
   D. Outcome statement

10. Select the meaning of the underlined word in the sentence.
    The child developed a <u>labile</u> condition that worried the parents, so they brought the child to the doctor's office for a checkup.
    A. Fevered
    B. Volatile
    C. Stomach
    D. Vision

11. The nurse noted in the chart, "The patient is lethargic." How was the patient behaving?
    A. Pacing the halls, yelling at the staff
    B. Difficult to arouse
    C. Shaking uncontrollably
    D. Not responding to painful stimuli

12. Select the meaning of the underlined word in the sentence.
    The doctor made an <u>initial</u> examination of the patient.
    A. Complete
    B. First
    C. Incomplete
    D. Discharge

13. Select the word or phrase that will identify the correct meaning of the underlined word.
    Progeny is a term used to describe a person's
    _____.
    A. creditors
    B. offspring
    C. hereditary disease
    D. health status

14. What is the best description for the word *distal*?
    A. The part of the heart that receives blood from the lungs
    B. Urgent
    C. The part of the body farthest from the injury
    D. Empathetic

15. Select the correct definition of the underlined word.
    The <u>incidence</u> of smoking has decreased in recent years because of the effectiveness of advertising campaigns.
    A. Prestige
    B. Glamour
    C. Occurrence
    D. Influence

16. Select the correct definition of the underlined word.
    The <u>symmetrical</u> nature of the artwork allowed it to be viewed from many angles.
    A. Measured from the center
    B. Colorful
    C. Equal on all sides
    D. Whimsical

17. Select the word or phrase that will make the sentence grammatically correct.
    Within the _____ of the hospital, great emphasis is placed on calmness.
    A. cafeteria
    B. milieu
    C. metabolism
    D. component

18. Select the correct definition of the underlined word.
    The <u>verbal</u> instructions given by the instructor allowed the student to create an outstanding project.
    A. Written
    B. Detailed
    C. Oral
    D. Permissive

19. What is the best description for the term *quotient*?
    A. The minimum number of members needed to be present for a vote to be valid
    B. The protocol used when a sterile field must be maintained
    C. A math term naming the answer in a division question
    D. The preferred inoculation site for a newborn infant

20. Select the word or phrase that will make the sentence grammatically correct.
The nurse has a _____ to the *Journal of Nursing Education.*
A. subscription
B. prescription
C. recipe
D. receipt

21. Select the word or phrase that will make the sentence grammatically correct.
The food bank referred many _____ patients to the free clinic.
A. indignant
B. wealthy
C. indigent
D. healthy

22. What is the best description for the word *laceration?*
A. The means by which nursing mothers produce milk for their babies
B. A deep, ragged tear
C. A medical term used to describe the removal of the tear ducts
D. An intolerance of dairy products

23. Which statement uses a euphemism?
A. The fireman bravely entered the burning building.
B. The nurse told the family, "I'm sorry, your father has passed away."
C. The orderly was laughing about the patient's vomiting episode.
D. Her husband was overjoyed when she told him she was pregnant.

24. What is another word for skull?
A. Spine
B. Ability
C. Cranium
D. Zygote

25. Select the meaning of the underlined word in the sentence.
In medicine, the desired outcome is recovery.
A. expected
B. analyzed
C. wished for
D. diagnosed

26. What is the best description for the term *triage?*
A. The stand with three legs used to support an IV pump
B. The order in which patients are to be treated
C. The physician's prescription for a drug to be taken three times a day
D. The shift for nursing duty beginning at 3 pm and ending at 11 pm

27. Select the meaning of the underlined word in the sentence.
His skin was unevenly pigmented by the disease.
A. Scarred
B. Spotted
C. Broken
D. Colored

28. Which word means "the thickness of a liquid"?
A. Viscosity
B. Zygote
C. Sublingual
D. Adhesion

29. Select the correct definition of the underlined word.
The gaping hole in the fence was an enticing lure for the curious toddler.
A. Narrow
B. Jagged
C. Painted
D. Wide open

30. What is the best description for the term *febrile?*
A. Mental incompetence
B. Having a fever
C. Pregnant
D. Having clogged sinuses

31. What is the best description for the word *contraction?*
A. Spasm
B. Decrease
C. Treaty
D. Moderate

32. Select the meaning of the underlined word in the sentence.
The nurse discussed the diet plan with the patient.
A. Regime
B. Regimen

C. Supposition

D. Substitution

33. What is the best description for the term *combination*?

A. Putting two or more things together

B. The beginning of a fire

C. The reason for an action

D. The change seen when a drug is administered

34. Decomposition is the process of enzymes digesting food. Another name for this process is _____.

A. degeneration

B. dialysis

C. lysis

D. lymph

35. Select the meaning of the underlined word in the sentence.

The nurse noticed an <u>audible</u> gurgle when doing a physical examination on the patient.

A. Observable

B. Spasmodic

C. Ominous

D. Perceptible

36. Select the meaning of the underlined word in the sentence.

The nurse observed that the skin around the sore was <u>inflamed</u>.

A. Blanched

B. Covered with a scab

C. Cool to the touch

D. Reddened

37. Select the meaning of the underlined word in the sentence.

The nurse gave instructions to the patient on the care of his <u>renal</u> disease.

A. Fatal

B. Kidney

C. Heart

D. Lung

38. Select the meaning of the underlined word in the sentence.

<u>Endogenous</u> factors were responsible for his illness.

A. Produced within the body

B. Produced outside the body

C. Polluting

D. Hemocratic

39. Which word is not spelled correctly in the context of the sentence?

The ICU nurse-manger wanted all staff to sign the letter complaining about working hours at the unit.

A. ICU

B. sign

C. manger

D. complaining

40. Select the meaning of the underlined word in the sentence.

When examined, the laboring mother was at 50% <u>dilation</u>.

A. Blood pressure

B. Cervical opening

C. Birth process

D. Exhumation

41. Which word is not spelled correctly in the context of this sentence?

The nurse went form room to room looking for the missing patient.

A. patient

B. form

C. nurse

D. missing

42. Select the meaning of the underlined word in the sentence.

To <u>alleviate</u> his pain, the nurse gave the patient a PRN medication.

A. Pinpoint

B. Relocate

C. Eradicate

D. Reduce

43. Select the meaning of the underlined word in the sentence.

Being <u>bilingual</u> is an advantage for a nurse.

A. Able to speak more than one language

B. Able to use either hand with equal skill and ease

C. Not squeamish when seeing blood

D. Can remember everything that is read

44. What is the best description for the term *fracture*?

A. Break

B. Brake

C. Cut
D. Cure

45. Which word is not spelled correctly in the context of the sentence?
The physician thought it was unecessary to explain the procedure.
A. physician
B. unecessary
C. explain
D. procedure

46. Select the meaning of the underlined word in the sentence.
Exogenous factors will affect the patient's well-being.
A. Produced outside the body
B. Produced within the body
C. Produced by the kidneys
D. Hereditary

47. To implement something is to
_____.
A. prevent it from occurring
B. emphasize the importance of
C. cause it to happen
D. follow from beginning to end

48. Posterior refers to which part of the body?
A. Topmost
B. Lowermost
C. Front
D. Back

49. Select the meaning of the underlined word in the sentence.
The precipitous change was considered a good thing.
A. Difficult
B. Abrupt
C. Gentle
D. Unanticipated

50. Select the meaning of the underlined word in the sentence.
His untoward actions during the admission process created a problem for the nurse.
A. Violent
B. Casual
C. Unseemly
D. Capricious

51. Select the meaning of the underlined word in the sentence.
The practical nurse is planning to administer a transdermal medication.
A. Applied directly to the skin
B. Injected just barely under the skin
C. Injected in the tissue just below the skin layer
D. Directly under the tongue

52. Select the meaning of the underlined word in the sentence.
The potent medication reduced the symptoms almost immediately.
A. Correct
B. Strong
C. Liquid
D. Tablet

53. Which word can be defined as a truth, a rule, or a law?
A. Prescription
B. Tort
C. Principle
D. Malpractice

54. Select the meaning of the underlined word in the sentence.
The proliferation of text messaging among teens has alarmed parents.
A. Increase
B. Summarization
C. Ambiance
D. Rampant

55. Select the meaning of the underlined word in the sentence.
It is important that the bandage remain intact.
A. Dry
B. Whole
C. Uncovered
D. Secure

56. Select the meaning of the underlined word in the sentence.
It is not wise to skimp on personal hygiene.
A. Measures contributing to cleanliness and good health
B. Financial resources available through the employment department
C. Insurance
D. Friendliness

57. The patient fractured the lateral portion of the hip bone, which is known as the _____.
   A. ilium
   B. ileum
   C. icterus
   D. ileus

58. Select the meaning of the underlined word in the sentence.
   The parameters of medical ethics require the nurse to report instances of suspected child abuse.
   A. Laws
   B. Limits
   C. Common sense
   D. Structure

59. Select the correct order of words to fit in the sentence structure.
   The nursing _____ put the Band-_____ on the wound to _____ the nurse.
   A. aid, aide, aide
   B. aide, aid, aid
   C. aid, aide, aid
   D. aide, aid, aide

60. A person who is ravenous is _____.
   A. generous
   B. outspoken
   C. friendly
   D. hungry

VOCABULARY PRACTICE TEST ANSWER KEY

1. C	31. A
2. D	32. B
3. B	33. A
4. B	34. C
5. D	35. D
6. A	36. D
7. A	37. B
8. A	38. A
9. D	39. C
10. B	40. B
11. B	41. B
12. B	42. D
13. B	43. A
14. C	44. A
15. C	45. B
16. C	46. A
17. B	47. C
18. C	48. D
19. C	49. B
20. A	50. C
21. C	51. A
22. B	52. B
23. B	53. C
24. C	54. A
25. C	55. B
26. B	56. A
27. D	57. A
28. A	58. B
29. D	59. B
30. B	60. D

GRAMMAR PRACTICE TEST

1. Select the best word for the blank in the following sentence.
   He was _____ by her kind words.
   A. affect
   B. effect
   C. effected
   D. affected

2. Which of the following sentences is grammatically incorrect?
   A. He performed well on the test.
   B. He performed good on the test.
   C. He performed poorly on the test.
   D. He performed adequately on the test.

3. In the following sentence, which is the dependent clause?
   We played a game while we waited, and then we had dinner.
   A. We played
   B. then we had dinner
   C. while we waited
   D. a game

4. Which of the following sentences is grammatically correct?
   A. She drove much farther than I did.
   B. The campus is further up the road.
   C. I will have to consider farther before making a decision.
   D. The hospital was further away than he thought.

5. Select the best word for the blank in the following sentence.
   He thought it was _____ than 3 miles to the hospital.
   A. further
   B. fewer
   C. bigger
   D. less

6. Select the best words for the blanks in the following sentence.
   The patient wanted to _____ down on the bed, but first she had to _____ her tray of food on the table.
   A. lie, lay
   B. lay, lie
   C. lie, laid
   D. lain, lying

7. Which word from the following sentence is a noun?
   The bird flew across the blue sky.
   A. across
   B. flew
   C. bird
   D. blue

8. Which word in the following sentence is a conjunction?
   The little girl wanted a cookie, but she didn't take one.
   A. little
   B. but
   C. take
   D. the

9. Which word in the following sentence is a direct object?
   The nurse helped the patient with the medication.
   A. helped
   B. nurse
   C. patient
   D. medication

10. Which word or phrase in the following sentence is a subject?
    The nurses went to the conference room.
    A. conference
    B. went to
    C. room
    D. nurses

11. Which of the following sentences is grammatically correct?
    A. Walking home from class, the students watched the snow begin to fall.
    B. Walking home from class, the snow began falling on the students.
    C. Walking home from class, snow fell on the students.
    D. Walking home from class, the students watched the snow fell.

12. Select the best word for the blank in the following sentence.
    The student sang well, but she danced
    _____.
    A. bad
    B. badly
    C. poor
    D. poorer

13. Which of the following sentences is grammatically correct?
    A. I wanted ice cream; he wanted cake.
    B. I wanted ice cream he wanted cake.
    C. I wanted ice cream, he wanted cake.
    D. I wanted ice cream but he wanted cake.

14. Select the best word for the blank in the following sentence.
    The college _____ he chose is in New York
    A. which
    B. that
    C. who
    D. what

15. Select the best word or words for the blank in the following sentence.
    The nurses, except for Henry, _____ in the conference room.
    A. waits
    B. is waiting
    C. are waiting
    D. was waiting

16. Select the best word for the blank in the following sentence.
    Not only the students but also the professor _____ stunned by the test results.
    A. was
    B. were
    C. are
    D. be

17. Which word in the following sentence is a preposition?
    The university lost power during the storm.
    A. lost
    B. during
    C. power
    D. the

18. Which word or phrase in the following sentence is the predicate?
    Everyone who attended the concert heard the conductor's announcement.
    A. the conductor's announcement
    B. everyone
    C. heard the conductor's announcement
    D. who attended

19. The following sentence contains which type of phrase?
    The patient was fit as a fiddle.
    A. sexist language
    B. profanity
    C. euphemism
    D. cliché

20. Select the best word for the blank in the following sentence.
    The pack of wolves _____ running through the forest.
    A. are
    B. were
    C. is
    D. be

21. Which of the following sentences is grammatically correct?
    A. This semester I am taking classes in Spanish chemistry, and biology.
    B. This semester I am taking classes in Spanish, chemistry, and biology.
    C. This semester I am taking classes in Spanish chemistry and biology.
    D. This semester I am taking classes in Spanish, chemistry and biology

22. Which of the following sentences is grammatically correct?
    A. The room was filled with the perfume of flowers (e.g., plant blossoms).
    B. The room was filled with the perfume (e.g., scent) of flowers.
    C. The room (e.g., enclosed space) was filled with the perfume of flowers.
    D. The room was filled with the perfume of flowers (e.g., roses, lilies, and irises).

23. Which word in the following sentence is grammatically incorrect?
    Dr. Jones, who all of the patients like, plays the piano well.
    A. who
    B. well
    C. plays
    D. like

24. Which of the following sentences contains a predicate adjective?
    A. My classes are for smart students.
    B. Smart students are in my classes.
    C. My smart students are in these classes.
    D. The students in my classes are smart.

25. Select the sentence that is grammatically correct.
    A. The nurse spoke to my sister and I about our mother's condition.
    B. The nurse spoke to my sister and me about our mother's condition.
    C. The nurse spoke to me and my sister about our mother's condition.
    D. The nurse spoke to I and my sister about our mother's condition.

26. Select the word or phrase that makes this sentence grammatically correct.
    She has always been afraid of _____ to the doctor.
    A. go
    B. to go
    C. going
    D. have gone

27. Select the word or phrase that makes this sentence grammatically correct.
    Every morning after a shower, I shave _____.
    A. me
    B. myself
    C. mine
    D. my

28. Select the word or phrase that makes this sentence grammatically correct.
    The patient was _____ cold, so he asked the nurse for another blanket.
    A. too
    B. not
    C. to
    D. so much

29. Select the word or phrase that will make the sentence grammatically correct.
    Because I want to go to the movies later, I am going _____ my homework now.
    A. to do
    B. doing
    C. be doing
    D. to doing

30. Select the word or phrase that makes this sentence grammatically correct.
    He sat _____ Holly and Mary on the bus.
    A. though
    B. through
    C. among
    D. between

31. Select the word or phrase in the sentence that is not used correctly.
    The data confirms that the patient is suffering from extreme anxiety, and a tranquilizing medication is immediately required.
    A. extreme anxiety
    B. confirms
    C. is
    D. immediately

32. Select the word or phrase that will make the sentence grammatically correct.
    The professor had a huge _____ of tests to grade.
    A. number
    B. amount
    C. aggregate
    D. stacks

33. Which word is used incorrectly in the following sentence?
    Will you learn me how to do origami?
    A. me
    B. will
    C. learn
    D. origami

34. Select the correct word for the blank in the following sentence.
    The members of the group _____ to be seated together.
    A. wanting
    B. want
    C. wants
    D. waiting

35. Select the correct word for the blank in the following sentence.
    The student completed the test _____.
    A. quite
    B. quick
    C. quitely
    D. quickly

36. Select the correct word(s) for the blank in the following sentence.
    The student thought the second test was _____ than the first test.
    A. harder
    B. more hard
    C. hardest
    D. most hardest

37. Select the correct word for the blank in the following sentence.
    The dog wagged _____ tail when the food dish was filled.
    A. the
    B. one's
    C. its
    D. it's

38. What word is best to substitute for the underlined words in the following sentence?
    The boy watched the lights in the house go off.
    A. Him
    B. His
    C. They
    D. He

39. Select the word or phrase that will make the sentence grammatically correct.
    _____ thought the movie was very good.
    A. Us
    B. We
    C. Them
    D. Ourselves

40. Select the word or phrase that makes this sentence grammatically correct.
    The hospital is located at the top _____ the hill.
    A. of
    B. off
    C. in
    D. on

GRAMMAR PRACTICE TEST ANSWER KEY

1.	D	21.	B
2.	B	22.	D
3.	C	23.	A
4.	A	24.	D
5.	D	25.	B
6.	A	26.	C
7.	C	27.	B
8.	B	28.	A
9.	C	29.	A
10.	D	30.	D
11.	A	31.	B
12.	B	32.	A
13.	A	33.	C
14.	B	34.	B
15.	C	35.	D
16.	A	36.	A
17.	B	37.	C
18.	C	38.	D
19.	D	39.	B
20.	C	40.	A

BIOLOGY PRACTICE TEST

1. In the hierarchic system of classification, which of the following is the least inclusive?
   A. Kingdom
   B. Class
   C. Genus
   D. Species

2. After observing an event, you develop an explanation. This statement is referred to as which of the following?
   A. Hypothesis
   B. Experiment
   C. Conclusion
   D. Theory

3. A molecule of water is bonded with another molecule of water by what type of bond?
   A. Ionic
   B. Covalent
   C. Hydrogen
   D. Molecular

4. Which of the following is a benefit of the intermolecular hydrogen bonding of water? (Select all that apply.)
   A. Water has a relatively high specific heat value.
   B. Water has strong cohesive and adhesive properties.
   C. Polarity of water allows it to act as a versatile solvent.
   D. Water moves from higher to lower concentrations.

5. Of all the molecules that are significant to biology, which of the following are considered the most important?
   A. Carbohydrates, lipids, protein, and nucleic acids
   B. Carbohydrates, lipids, protein, and calcium
   C. Carbohydrates, lipids, protein, and sulfur
   D. Carbohydrates, lipids, protein, and iron

6. Lipids are better known as fats, but what are they specifically? (Select all that apply.)
   A. Fatty acids
   B. Phospholipids
   C. Ketones
   D. Steroids

7. What are the two categories of fatty acids?
   A. Trans fat and saturated fats
   B. Trans fat and unsaturated fats
   C. Saturated fats and unsaturated fats
   D. Saturated fats and polyunsaturated fats

8. How do phospholipids function in cells?
   A. They are integral components of the nuclear membrane.
   B. They are integral components of the cytoplasmic skeleton.
   C. They are integral components of the mitochondrial membranes.
   D. They are integral components of the plasma membrane.

9. Which of the biologic molecules are considered the most significant contributor to cellular function?
   A. Carbohydrates
   B. Lipids
   C. Proteins
   D. Nucleic acids

10. Proteins are polymers of which of the following?
    A. Monosaccharides
    B. Amino acids
    C. Fatty acids
    D. Nucleotides

11. Which of the following proteins catalyze different reactions or processes?
    A. Keratin
    B. Hormone
    C. Enzyme
    D. Collagen

12. Which of the biologic molecules are components of the molecules of inheritance?
    A. Carbohydrates
    B. Lipids
    C. Proteins
    D. Nucleic acids

13. What is the sum of all chemical reactions that occur in an organism?
    A. Catalysis
    B. Metabolism
    C. Catabolism
    D. Anabolism

14. In a cell, reactions take place in a series of steps called:
    A. Metabolic pathways
    B. Chemical bonding
    C. Synthesis
    D. Hydrolysis

15. What is the fundamental unit of biology?
    A. Atom
    B. Cell
    C. Tissue
    D. Organ

16. Which type of cell contains no defined nucleus?
    A. Prokaryotic cell
    B. Eukaryotic cell
    C. Animal cell
    D. Protest cell

17. What is the primary purpose of the flagella on the surface of cells?
    A. Movement of the cell
    B. Removal of cellular waste
    C. Replication of chromosomes
    D. Production of energy

18. Which cell organelle functions to transport materials from the endoplasmic reticulum throughout the cell?
    A. Ribosome
    B. Golgi apparatus
    C. Lysosome
    D. Vacuole

19. Which of the following are the distinct organelles that produce cell energy?
    A. Mitochondrion and chloroplast
    B. Mitochondrion and nucleus
    C. Chloroplast and nucleus
    D. Chloroplast and lysosome

20. Which component of the cell contributes to the protection, communication, and passage of substances into and out of the cell?
    A. Nucleus
    B. Cell membrane
    C. Endoplasmic reticulum
    D. Cytoplasm

21. The cell membrane consists of a bilayer of phospholipids with proteins, cholesterol, and glycoproteins. This bilayer creates a hydrophobic region between two layers of lipids, making it which of the following?
    A. Impermeable
    B. Permeable
    C. Selectively permeable
    D. Selectively impermeable

22. What are the two catabolic pathways that lead to cellular energy production?
    A. Fermentation and internal respiration
    B. Fermentation and external respiration
    C. Fermentation and cellular respiration
    D. Fermentation and anaerobic respiration

23. What is the first step in the conversion of glucose to pyruvate?
    A. Glycolysis
    B. Krebs cycle
    C. Electron transport chain
    D. Aerobic respiration

24. Which step in cellular respiration yields the greatest amount of ATP?
    A. Glycolysis
    B. Krebs cycle
    C. Electron transport chain
    D. Fermentation

25. During cell respiration, the conversion of glucose results in an overall production of how many ATP molecules?
    A. 2
    B. 16
    C. 18-24
    D. 32-36

26. What is the function of water in photosynthesis?
    A. Combine with carbon dioxide
    B. Absorb light energy
    C. Supply electrons in the light reactions
    D. Transport hydrogen ions in the dark reactions

27. Cells reproduce by different processes, all of which fall into what two categories?
    A. Sexual reproduction and binary fission
    B. Sexual reproduction and asexual reproduction
    C. Asexual reproduction and binary fission
    D. Asexual reproduction and mitosis

28. Which of the following describes how a bacterium reproduces?
    A. Mitosis
    B. Meiosis
    C. Binary fission
    D. Cytokinesis

29. Regarding mitosis and cytokinesis, one difference between higher plants and animals is that in plants:
    A. The spindles contain cellulose microfibrils in addition to microtubules, whereas animal spindles do not contain microfibrils.
    B. Sister chromatids are identical, whereas in animals they differ from one another.
    C. A cell plate begins to form at telophase, whereas in animals a cleavage furrow is initiated at that stage.
    D. Chromosomes become attached to the spindle at prophase, whereas in animals chromosomes do not become attached until anaphase.

30. During which phase of cell reproduction does the cell divide forming two separate identical cells?
    A. Prophase
    B. Metaphase
    C. Anaphase
    D. Cytokinesis

31. How does meiosis differ from mitosis?
    A. In meiosis, each of the daughter cells contains twice as many chromosomes as the parent.
    B. In meiosis, each of the daughter cells contains half as many chromosomes as the parent.
    C. In meiosis, each of the daughter cells is completely identical to the parent.
    D. Meiotic division occurs in all body cells, whereas in mitosis the cells only divide in the gonads.

32. At which phase of meiosis does crossing over occur?
    A. Prophase I
    B. Prophase II
    C. Metaphase I
    D. Metaphase II

33. A cell division occurs in a human. The resulting cells contain 23 chromosomes. This is a description of gametes formed by which process?
    A. Mitosis
    B. Binary fission
    C. Meiosis
    D. Cytokinesis

34. If you wanted to determine the probability of a genotype, which of the following would you use?
A. Karyotype
B. Electrophoresis
C. Punnett square
D. Genotype map

35. Which of the following terms is used to describe the appearance of the organism?
A. Homozygous
B. Heterozygous
C. Phenotype
D. Genotype

36. What is the probability that a recessive trait would be expressed in offspring if two parents who are both heterozygous for the desired trait were crossed?
A. 100%
B. 75%
C. 50%
D. 25%

37. Because genetics is the study of heredity, many human disorders can be determined by studying a person's chromosomes or by creating which of the following?
A. Punnett square
B. Pedigree
C. Chromosome model
D. Genetic map

38. Why is DNA important for metabolic activities of the cell?
A. It initiates cellular mitosis.
B. It provides cell wall stability.
C. It increases glucose absorption.
D. It controls the synthesis of enzymes.

39. During protein synthesis, what process uses an RNA strand to produce a complementary strand of DNA?
A. Transcription
B. Translation
C. Transfer synthesis
D. Codon synthesis

40. During the process of transcription, a sequence of RNA is generated in which the RNA base cytosine (C) is inserted complementary to the DNA base guanine (G). Which RNA base is inserted complementary to the DNA base thymine (T)?
A. Adenine
B. Cytosine
C. Quinine
D. Thymine

BIOLOGY PRACTICE TEST ANSWER KEY

1. D
2. A
3. C
4. A, B, C
5. A
6. A, B, D
7. C
8. D
9. C
10. B
11. C
12. D
13. B
14. A
15. B
16. A
17. A
18. B
19. A
20. B

21. C
22. C
23. A
24. C
25. D
26. C
27. B
28. C
29. C
30. D
31. B
32. A
33. C
34. C
35. C
36. D
37. B
38. D
39. A
40. A

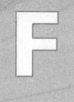
CHEMISTRY PRACTICE TEST

1. What are all metric measurements composed of?
   A. Metric prefix and a basic unit of measure
   B. A significand and a metric prefix
   C. A metric prefix and a coefficient
   D. A coefficient and a significand

2. What is the most *commonly* used temperature scale in the scientific community?
   A. Fahrenheit
   B. Celsius or Centigrade
   C. Kelvin
   D. English temperature method

3. The nucleus of an atom contains or is made up of which of the following?
   A. Protons and electrons
   B. Protons only
   C. Protons and neutrons
   D. Neutrons and electrons

4. What is an atom that has a positive charge called?
   A. A cathode
   B. A cation
   C. An anode
   D. An anion

5. In the periodic table, what are the rows called?
   A. Groups
   B. Moles
   C. Columns
   D. Periods

6. What is the atomic number?
   A. Number of neutrons
   B. Number of protons
   C. Number of electrons
   D. Number of isotopes

7. Which of the following describes the atomic mass?
   A. Mass of protons and electrons
   B. Mass of neutrons and electrons
   C. Average mass of that element's isotopes
   D. Number of moles in a solution

8. Chemical equations are written in which manner?
   A. Product → Reactants
   B. Reactants → Products
   C. Reactants + Reactants
   D. Products + Reactants

9. What is the charge on potassium in the compound KCl?
   A. −1
   B. +1
   C. −2
   D. +2

10. A catalyst is a substance that accelerates a reaction by which of the following?
    A. Adding energy to the overall reaction
    B. Increasing the amount of energy needed for the reaction to occur
    C. Finding an alternate pathway for a reaction that requires less energy
    D. Speeding up the overall reaction process

11. Percent concentration of a solution is expressed as which of the following?
    A. 100 parts per 100 dL
    B. Parts per 100 parts
    C. Parts of moles
    D. Moles per 100 parts

12. What will one liter of a one molar solution of any element contain?
    A. The atomic mass in grams of that element
    B. The atomic number in grams of that element
    C. The atomic mass in liters of that element
    D. The atomic number in liters of that element

13. Chemical bonding is the bonding of which of the following?
    A. One atom to another atom
    B. One mole to another mole
    C. A proton to an electron
    D. One cation to another cation

14. Which of the following describes an ionic bond?
    A. It shares electrons.
    B. It does not share electrons.
    C. It is sometimes called a covalent bond.
    D. It is the strongest of all chemical bonds.

15. The reaction $2C_2H_6 + 7O_2 \rightarrow 4CO_2 + 6H_2O$ has a ratio of 2 parts ethane (C_2H_6) and 7 parts oxygen (O_2). How many parts of ethane (C_2H_6) will be needed to react with 21 parts of oxygen (O_2)?
    A. 3 parts of ethane C_2H_6
    B. 6 parts of ethane C_2H_6
    C. 9 parts of ethane C_2H_6
    D. 14 parts of ethane C_2H_6

16. What is the concentration of 58.5 g of NaCl in 2 L of solution (atomic weights of each element are as follows: Na = 23 g/mol, Cl = 35.5 g/mol)?
    A. 0.5 mol NaCl
    B. 0.75 mol NaCl
    C. 1 mol NaCl
    D. 2 mol NaCl

17. In a redox reaction, which of the following describes reduction?
    A. It is the loss of electrons.
    B. It is the gain of protons.
    C. It is the loss of a neutron.
    D. It is the gain of electrons.

18. What are acids?
    A. Hydrogen acceptors
    B. Solutions of high pH
    C. Hydrogen donors
    D. Amphoteric

19. What is a benefit of water's ability to make hydrogen bonds?
    A. Lack of cohesiveness
    B. Low surface tension
    C. Use as a nonpolar solvent
    D. High specific heat

20. What are bases or alkaline solutions?
    A. Hydrogen acceptors
    B. Solutions of low pH
    C. Hydrogen donors
    D. Amphoteric

21. Chemical reactions in living systems proceed along catabolic pathways, and there tends to be an increase in which of the following?
    A. Entropy
    B. Enthalpy
    C. Glucose
    D. Glycogen

22. What is a pH of 7?
    A. Acidic
    B. Basic
    C. Neutral
    D. Positive

23. Which is the correct way to write Iodine (I) with an atomic mass of 131?
    A. I^{131}
    B. I_{131}
    C. ^{131}I
    D. $_{131}I$

24. What is the correct formula for magnesium chloride?
    A. $MgCl_2$
    B. $MgCl$
    C. Mg_2Cl
    D. Mg_2Cl_2

25. What is the weakest of all the intermolecular forces?
    A. Dispersion
    B. Dipole interactions
    C. Hydrogen bonding
    D. Covalent bonding

26. Beta radiation is the emission of which of the following?
    A. Large numbers of helium ions
    B. An electron
    C. High energy electromagnetic radiation
    D. A product of the decomposition of a proton

27. Which of the following describes carbohydrates?
    A. They serve as fuel for the body.
    B. They are present in DNA but not in RNA.
    C. They are the least abundant biomolecule.
    D. They cannot be stored in the body.

28. What are monosaccharides?
    A. The simplest form of carbohydrates
    B. The most complex form of carbohydrates
    C. One form of a very complex fat
    D. Artificial sweeteners such as saccharin

29. Disaccharides are the joining together of which of the following?
    A. Three to six monosaccharides
    B. Two monosaccharides
    C. A number of monosaccharides
    D. A fat and a monosaccharide

30. Glycolysis is one of the body's chemical pathways for which of the following?
    A. Manufacturing glycogen
    B. Building proteins
    C. Producing fats
    D. Metabolizing glucose

31. Amino acids are the building blocks for which of the following?
    A. Nucleic acids
    B. Carbohydrates
    C. Proteins
    D. Lipids

32. What is the union of two amino acids using a peptide bond called?
    A. A dipeptide
    B. A peptide
    C. A monopeptide
    D. A polypeptide

33. Which of the following describes lipids?
    A. They are a major source of fuel for the body immediately after a meal.
    B. They are stored for a source of fuel after carbohydrate depletion.
    C. They are comprised of glycerol and three fatty acids.
    D. They are metabolized by a pathway called glycolysis.

34. Which of the following describes DNA?
    A. It is made of two strands of a ribose sugar-phosphate chain.
    B. It consists of two strands of a deoxyribose sugar-phosphate chain.
    C. It consists of one strand of a ribose sugar-phosphate chain.
    D. It is located solely in the mitochondria of individual cells.

35. Use of the periodic table allows prediction of which of the following?
    A. The properties of each of the elements
    B. The charge of polyatomic ions
    C. The number of isotopes in each element
    D. The potential for discovery of new elements

36. How could water be boiled at room temperature?
    A. By lowering the pressure
    B. By increasing the pressure
    C. By decreasing the volume
    D. By raising the boiling point

37. What is a combustion reaction?
  A. It is endothermic.
  B. It substitutes one element for another.
  C. It always shares electrons.
  D. It is a reaction that involves oxygen.

38. What is $KCl \rightarrow K + Cl_2$ an example of?
  A. Synthesis
  B. Decomposition
  C. Single replacement
  D. Double replacement

39. Iodine and carbon dioxide undergo sublimation at room temperature and atmospheric pressure. What is this process?
  A. Changing from a gas to a solid
  B. Changing from a liquid to a gas
  C. Changing from a solid to a liquid
  D. Changing from a solid to a gas

40. An experiment is performed to measure the temperature of boiling water at sea level. The actual boiling point is 104.6° C, 104.5° C, and 104.4° C. What term best describes these data?
  A. Accurate
  B. Precise
  C. Variable
  D. Equivalent

CHEMISTRY PRACTICE TEST ANSWER KEY

1. A		**21.** A	
2. B		**22.** C	
3. C		**23.** C	
4. B		**24.** A	
5. D		**25.** A	
6. B		**26.** B	
7. C		**27.** A	
8. B		**28.** A	
9. B		**29.** B	
10. C		**30.** D	
11. B		**31.** C	
12. A		**32.** A	
13. A		**33.** B	
14. B		**34.** B	
15. B		**35.** A	
16. A		**36.** A	
17. D		**37.** D	
18. C		**38.** B	
19. D		**39.** D	
20. A		**40.** B	

ANATOMY AND PHYSIOLOGY PRACTICE TEST

1. What mineral is responsible for muscle contractions?
   A. Chloride
   B. Sodium
   C. Calcium
   D. Magnesium

2. In which of the following locations would the urinary bladder and internal reproductive organs be found?
   A. Thoracic cavity
   B. Mediastinum
   C. Abdominal cavity
   D. Pelvic cavity

3. What separates the thoracic cavity from the abdominal cavity?
   A. Diaphragm
   B. Mediastinum
   C. Liver
   D. Lungs

4. Which of the following epithelial types is correctly matched with its major function?
   A. Simple squamous epithelium—secretion or absorption
   B. Stratified squamous epithelium—changes shape when stretched
   C. Stratified squamous epithelium—diffusion
   D. Simple columnar epithelium—secretion or absorption

5. A tissue examined under the microscope exhibits the following characteristics: cells found on internal surface of stomach, no extracellular matrix, cells tall and thin, no blood vessels in the tissue. What type of tissue is this?
   A. Epithelial
   B. Connective
   C. Muscle
   D. Cartilage
   E. Nervous

6. Nerve tissue is composed of neurons and connective tissue cells that are referred to as which of the following?
   A. Osteoblasts
   B. Neuroglia
   C. Osteocytes
   D. Arterioles

7. Which tissue serves as the framework of the body by providing support and structure for the organs?
   A. Epithelial
   B. Connective
   C. Nervous
   D. Muscle

8. What is the basic unit of life and the building block of tissues and organs?
   A. Atom
   B. Organelle
   C. Cell
   D. DNA

9. Which type of cell division takes place in the gonads?
   A. Mitosis
   B. Meiosis
   C. Binary fission
   D. Asexual division

10. In what area of the body would you expect to find an especially thick stratum corneum?
    A. Back of the hand
    B. Heel of the foot
    C. Abdomen
    D. Over the shin

11. What are the glands of skin that produce a thin, watery secretion?
    A. Sebaceous glands
    B. Eccrine glands
    C. Apocrine glands
    D. Endocrine glands

12. Skin aids in maintaining the calcium and phosphate levels of the body by participating in the production of which of the following?
    A. Sebum
    B. Keratin
    C. Vitamin A
    D. Vitamin D

13. Which of the following are functions of the skeletal system? (Select all that apply.)
    A. Support the body
    B. Hemopoiesis
    C. Conduct impulses
    D. Provide protection

14. The orthopedic surgeon informs you that you have broken the middle region of the humerus. What is he describing?
    A. Epiphysis
    B. Articular cartilage
    C. Perichondrium
    D. Diaphysis

15. You have been given a sample of tissue that has open spaces partially filled by an assemblage of needlelike structures. What is the tissue?
    A. Spongy bone
    B. Compact bone
    C. Cartilage
    D. Adipose tissue

16. Which of the following bones is the only moveable bone of the skull?
    A. Maxilla
    B. Zygomatic
    C. Lacrimal
    D. Mandible

17. Which mineral is responsible for regulating fluid in the body?
    A. Chloride
    B. Sodium
    C. Calcium
    D. Magnesium

18. Why are skeletal muscles also called voluntary muscles?
    A. They are under conscious control.
    B. They are attached to the skeleton.
    C. They use ATP to energize contraction.
    D. They are striated in appearance.

19. All actions of the nervous system depend on the transmission of nerve impulses over which of the following?
    A. Neuroglia
    B. Efferent pathways
    C. Afferent pathways
    D. Neurons

20. Motor or _____ neurons transmit nerve impulses away from the CNS.
    A. Afferent
    B. Efferent
    C. Central
    D. Peripheral

21. Jeffery has contracted bulbar poliomyelitis, and it has affected the medulla oblongata. The doctors warned the family that his condition is grave and death may be imminent. What functions of the medulla oblongata have warranted such a dire prognosis?
    A. The medulla oblongata contains vital centers that control heart action, blood vessel diameter, and respiration.
    B. The medulla oblongata contains neural connections of the reticular-activating system.
    C. The medulla oblongata contains the pineal gland, which controls the vital centers.
    D. The medulla oblongata contains the corpora quadrigemina, which controls the neural transmission of impulses along the spinal cord.

22. What are chemical messengers that control growth, differentiation, and the metabolism of specific target cells called?
    A. Hormones
    B. Neurons
    C. Glands
    D. Second messengers

23. Which of the following are tropic hormones? (Select all that apply.)
    A. Somatotropin
    B. Follicle-stimulating hormone
    C. Antidiuretic hormone
    D. Thyroid-stimulating hormone

24. Which leukocytes are correctly matched with their function or description? (Select all that apply.)
    A. Monocytes—become macrophages
    B. Basophils—the most common type of WBC
    C. Lymphocytes—important in immune response
    D. Neutrophils—phagocytize microorganisms

25. The heart has an intrinsic beat that is initiated by which of the following?
    A. Semilunar valve
    B. Bicuspid valve
    C. Tricuspid valve
    D. Sinoatrial node

26. Vasodilation and vasoconstriction result from which of the following?
    A. Contraction of smooth muscle in the arterial wall
    B. Relaxation of smooth muscle in the arterial wall
    C. Relaxation and contraction of smooth muscle in the arterial wall
    D. Contraction and relaxation of smooth muscle in the venous wall

27. Which of the following is the blood vessel where exchanges take place between blood and the cells of the body?
    A. Artery
    B. Vein
    C. Capillary
    D. Arteriole

28. What is the exchange of gases between the atmosphere and the blood through the alveoli called?
    A. External respiration
    B. Internal respiration
    C. Inhalation
    D. Cellular respiration

29. In order for inhalation to occur, what must happen?
    A. Contraction of the diaphragm, which decreases the volume of the chest cavity and draws air into the lungs
    B. Contraction of the diaphragm, which enlarges the chest cavity and draws air into the lungs
    C. Recoil of the lungs as the respiratory muscles contract, and the thorax decreases in size
    D. Recoil of the lungs as the respiratory muscles relax, and the thorax decreases in size

30. Most of the carbon dioxide in the blood does which of the following?
    A. It is carried in solution or bound to blood proteins.
    B. It is carried on hemoglobin.
    C. It is converted to bicarbonate ions by carbonic anhydrase within red blood cells.
    D. It is converted to bicarbonate ions by carbonic anhydrase within the plasma.

31. How does the trachea remain open like a hollow tube?
    A. Air pressure inside keeps it open.
    B. Supporting cartilaginous rings keep it open.
    C. It is reinforced with bone that cannot collapse.
    D. Special muscles are working to keep the trachea open.

32. The stomach muscle churns and mixes food, turning the mass into a soupy substance called which of the following?
    A. Bolus
    B. Bile
    C. Chyme
    D. Feces

33. What is the function of aldosterone?
    A. It converts proinsulin to insulin.
    B. It conserves sodium in the body.
    C. It protects against stress.
    D. It affects heat production.

34. All the nutrients that enter the hepatic portal vein are routed where for decontamination?
    A. Kidney
    B. Pancreas
    C. Spleen
    D. Liver

35. Which are the functional units of the kidney?
    A. Ureters
    B. Glomeruli
    C. Nephrons
    D. Renal capsules

36. What are the two functions of the male and female sex organs?
    A. Production of all cells and production of hormones
    B. Production of interstitial cells and production of hormones
    C. Production of gametes and production of hormones
    D. Production of gametes and production of interstitial cells

37. In men, spermatozoa develop within the _____ of each testis.
    A. Seminiferous tubules
    B. Vas deferens
    C. Ejaculatory ducts
    D. Bulbourethral glands

38. Testicular activity is under the control of which hormone(s)?
    A. FSH
    B. LH
    C. GH
    D. Both FSH and LH

39. Which hormone initiates the preparation of the endometrium of the uterus for pregnancy?
    A. FSH
    B. Estrogen
    C. LH
    D. Progesterone

40. During pregnancy, what organ produces the hormones that maintain the endometrium and prepare the breasts for milk production?
    A. Placenta
    B. Uterus
    C. Cervix
    D. Corpus luteum

ANATOMY AND PHYSIOLOGY PRACTICE TEST ANSWER KEY

1. C
2. D
3. A
4. D
5. A
6. B
7. B
8. C
9. B
10. B
11. B
12. D
13. A, B, D
14. D
15. A
16. D
17. B
18. A
19. D
20. B

21. A
22. A
23. A, B, D
24. A, C, D
25. D
26. C
27. C
28. A
29. B
30. C
31. B
32. C
33. B
34. D
35. C
36. C
37. A
38. D
39. B
40. A

PHYSICS PRACTICE TEST

1. Which physical quantity is scalar in nature?
   A. 3:42 PM
   B. 23 m/sec; east
   C. 723 Nm; 216 degrees
   D. 34 km/sec; sin (120 degrees)

2. A bicycle trip of 680 m takes 12.6 seconds. What is the average speed of the bicycle?
   A. 53.97 m/sec
   B. 8,568 m/sec
   C. 0.054 km/min
   D. 8.57 m/sec

3. A go-cart has an initial speed of 23.4 m/sec. Fifteen seconds later the go-cart has a final speed of 46.8 m/sec. What is the magnitude of the go-cart's acceleration?
   A. 702 m/sec^2
   B. 1.56 m/sec^2
   C. 362.7 m/sec^2
   D. 2.56 m/sec^2

4. You walk for 15 minutes at 3.8 m/sec and then decide to run for 12 minutes at 2.5 m/sec. What is your average speed?
   A. 3.22 m/sec
   B. 3.15 m/sec
   C. 13.5 m/sec
   D. 1.125 m/sec

5. A cannon is placed on the edge of a cliff that is 300 m tall. The barrel of the cannon is parallel to the ground below. If a cannonball leaves the barrel in a horizontal direction with a velocity of 115 m/sec, how far out from the base of the cliff will the cannonball land?
   A. 450.0 m
   B. 630.0 m
   C. 900.0 m
   D. 7,040.3 m

6. An object has a mass of 1,285 g. Determine the weight of the object in newtons.
   A. 12,593 N
   B. 125.93 N
   C. 12.59 N
   D. 1,259.3 N

7. A car that weighs 15,000 N is initially moving at 60 km/hr when the brakes are applied. The car is brought to a stop in 30 m. Assuming the force applied by the brakes is constant, determine the magnitude of the braking force.
   A. 7,086.7 N
   B. 900,000 N
   C. 1,500,000 N
   D. 30,000 N

8. A hockey puck of mass 0.450 kg is sliding across the ice. The puck is initially moving at 28 m/sec. However, because of the frictional force between the puck and the ice, the motion of the puck is stopped in 15.8 seconds. Determine the magnitude of the frictional force.
   A. 1.65 N
   B. 7.81 N
   C. 0.80 N
   D. 5.49 N

9. A race car has an initial velocity of 200 m/sec and over 4 seconds its velocity increases to 1200 m/sec. What is its acceleration?
   A. 100 m/sec^2
   B. 150 m/sec^2
   C. 200 m/sec^2
   D. 250 m/sec^2

10. What is the kinetic energy of a 1,200-kg roadster moving at a rate of 88 km/hr?
    A. 9,292,800 J
    B. 105,600 J
    C. 358,519 J
    D. 52,800 J

11. An archer exerts a force of 15 N to pull back the bowstring 15 cm as she prepares to shoot an arrow. How much kinetic energy will be imparted to the arrow as a result of the work done?
    A. 225 J
    B. 112.5 J
    C. 2.25 J
    D. 1.125 J

12. A book with a mass of 0.95 kg is held 2.3 m above the ground. Determine the gravitational potential energy of the book.
    A. 21.41 J
    B. 10.71 J
    C. 29.8 J
    D. 69.92 J

13. A 1,250-kg truck has a velocity of 28 m/sec to the east. What is the momentum of the truck?
    A. 17,500 kg-m/sec; east
    B. 35,000 kg-m/sec; west
    C. 35,000 kg-m/sec; east
    D. 17,500 kg-m/sec; west

14. A car of mass 1,350 kg experiences a force of 1500 N for 20 seconds. Determine the change in magnitude of the car's momentum.
    A. 15,000 N-sec
    B. 30,000 kg-m/sec
    C. 227,000 N-sec
    D. 101,250 kg-m/sec

15. A pendulum makes 12 vibrations every 60 seconds. What is the frequency of the pendulum?
    A. 5 Hz
    B. 0.083333 Hz
    C. 0.2 Hz
    D. 10 Hz

16. Three resistors are placed in series. The resistors have values of 110 ohms, 45 ohms, and 60 ohms. Determine the value of the voltage needed to provide a current of 2 amp to this set of series resistors.
    A. 430 V
    B. 220 V
    C. 210 V
    D. 107.5 V

17. Electric fields are vector quantities because they are completely described by both magnitude and direction. According to scientific convention, the direction of an electric field is which of the following?
    A. Away from a positive charge.
    B. Toward a positive charge.
    C. The direction a negative test charge would move when placed in an electric field.
    D. Away from a negative charge.

18. When a concave mirror is used, where would an enlarged, virtual image be formed?
    A. At the focal point of the mirror
    B. Between the focal point and the mirror
    C. Behind the mirror
    D. At the center of curvature of the mirror

19. A certain ocean wave has a frequency of 0.05 Hz and a wavelength of 10 m. What is the wave's speed?
    A. 0.5 m/sec
    B. 200 m/sec
    C. 0.005 m/sec
    D. 100 m/sec

20. Sound is an example of _____.
    A. a longitudinal wave
    B. a transverse wave
    C. a standing wave
    D. a Doppler wave

21. An object has a weight of 6,000 N when resting on the surface of the Earth. When located at a distance that is 3.2×10^7 m from the center of the Earth, what is the new weight of the object? Remember that the radius of the Earth is 6.4×10^6 m and the mass of the Earth is 6×10^{24} kg.
    A. 120 N
    B. 240 N
    C. 30,000 N
    D. 150,000 N

22. Which of the following must be known to calculate average speed?
    A. Distance and direction only
    B. Direction and velocity only
    C. Velocity and time only
    D. Distance and time

23. When calculating projectile motion, the horizontal motion is a function of which of the following?
    A. Distance and direction only
    B. Direction and velocity only
    C. Velocity and time only
    D. Distance and time

24. Which of the following values represents a balance force?
    A. 30 N east and 27 N west
    B. 500 N left and 500 N right
    C. 25 N up and 20 N down
    D. 1000 N north and 1200 N south

25. The upward force of air on an object is 30 N, and the downward force of gravity on the same object is 20 N. What is the net force?
    A. 10 N
    B. 50 N
    C. 1.5 N
    D. 0 N

26. What is the force necessary to move a 12-kg box at a rate of 10 m/sec^2?
    A. 12 N
    B. 10 N
    C. 200 N
    D. 120 N

27. Which of the following is an example of an electromagnetic wave?
    A. Radiowave
    B. Water wave
    C. Seismic wave
    D. Sound wave

28. A wave has a frequency of 15 Hz and a speed of 20 m/sec. What is its wavelength?
    A. 0.2 m
    B. 1.0 m
    C. 1.3 m
    D. 2.2 m

29. What is the speed of a wave with a frequency of 30 Hz and a wavelength of 0.7 m?
    A. 15 m/sec
    B. 21 m/sec
    C. 27 m/sec
    D. 32 m/sec

30. As a light wave enters a slower medium, what happens in terms of refraction related to normal?
    A. No change with regards to refraction.
    B. It will refract away from normal.
    C. It will refract toward normal.
    D. Light will not pass into a slower medium.

31. Which energy shell of an atom exhibits the greatest binding energy?
    A. K
    B. L
    C. M
    D. N

32. If an atom contains 14 protons in its nucleus, how many electrons must it contain to be stable?
    A. 11
    B. 12
    C. 13
    D. 14

33. What is the voltage in a circuit with a resistance of 2 ohms and a current of 55 amperes?
    A. 27.5 V
    B. 110 V
    C. 53 V
    D. 57 V

34. What is the resistance in a circuit with a current of 15 amperes and a voltage of 440 V?
    A. 455 ohms
    B. 425 ohms
    C. 29.3 ohms
    D. 6600 ohms

35. Pairs of magnets are placed in proximity to each other as below. Which pair will experience the greatest force of attraction?
    A. 0.5 T (north end) 1 meter from 0.5 T (north end)

    B. 2.5 T (south end) 1 meter from 0.5 T (south end)
    C. 2.5 T (south end) 1 meter from 0.5 T (north end)
    D. 2.5 T (north end) 1 meter from 2.5 T (south end)

PHYSICS PRACTICE TEST ANSWER KEY

1. A		19. A	
2. A		20. A	
3. B		21. B	
4. A		22. D	
5. C		23. C	
6. C		24. B	
7. A		25. A	
8. C		26. D	
9. D		27. A	
10. C		28. C	
11. C		29. B	
12. A		30. C	
13. C		31. A	
14. B		32. D	
15. C		33. B	
16. A		34. C	
17. A		35. D	
18. C			

GLOSSARY

A

Abstract noun The name of a quality or a general idea (e.g., persistence, democracy).

Acceleration The rate of change in velocity over a period of time.

Acid A compound that is a hydrogen or proton donor. It is corrosive to metals, changes blue litmus paper red, and becomes less acidic when mixed with bases.

Adjective A word, phrase, or clause that modifies a noun (the *biology* book) or pronoun (He is *nice*.).

Adverb A word, phrase, or clause that modifies a verb, an adjective, or another adverb.

Alimentary canal The digestive tube that consists of the mouth, pharynx, esophagus, stomach, small intestine, large intestine, rectum, and anus

Alleles Alternate versions of a gene.

Amino acids Organic compounds that contain at least one amino group and a carboxyl group; building blocks of proteins.

Amylase An enzyme in saliva.

Anatomic position. The position of the body where the body is erect, the feet are slightly apart, the head is held high, and the palms of the hands are facing forward.

Anterior View facing forward.

Antonym A word that means the opposite of another word.

Appendicular skeleton The part of the skeleton that includes the girdles and the limbs. The upper portion consists of the pectoral or shoulder girdle, the clavicle and scapula, and the upper extremity. The bones of the arm are the humerus, the radius and ulna, the carpals (wrist bones), the metacarpals (bones of the hand), and the phalanges (bones of the fingers). The lower portion of the appendicular skeleton is made up of the pelvic girdle or os coxae. Each of the os coxae consists of a fused ilium, ischium, and pubis. Bones of the lower extremity include the femur (thighbone), the tibia and fibula, the tarsals (ankle bones), the metatarsals (bones of the foot), and the phalanges.

Arterioles The smallest type of arteries.

Atom The basic building block of a molecule that contains a nucleus and orbits.

Atomic mass The *average* mass of each of that element's isotopes.

Atomic number The number of protons in the nucleus, and it defines an atom of a particular element.

Average speed The distance an object travels divided by the time the object travels without regard to direction of travel.

Axial skeleton The 28 bones of the skull. These are separated into the 14 facial bones and the 14 bones of the cranium.

B

Base A hydrogen or proton acceptor and generally has a hydroxide (OH) group in the makeup of the molecule. Bases are also called *alkaline compounds* and are substances that denature proteins, making them feel very slick; they change red litmus paper blue and become less basic when mixed with acids.

Basic unit of measure Standard unit of a system by which a quantity is accounted for and expressed (grams, liters, or meters).

Binary fission Type of asexual reproduction; parent cell splits into two identical daughter cells.

Binding energy How tightly the electron is bound to the nucleus.

Biochemistry The study of chemical processes in living organisms.

Bolus A ball of food that is formed after the food is broken down by the teeth and saliva.

C

Catalysts Substances that accelerate a reaction by reducing the activation energy or the amount of energy necessary for a reaction to occur.

Cell The basic unit of life and the building block of tissues and organs.

Celsius A temperature system used in most of the world and by the scientific community; abbreviated C. It has these characteristics: zero degrees (0° C) is the freezing point of pure water at sea level, and 100° C is the boiling point of pure water at sea level. Most people have a body temperature of 37° C.

Centripetal acceleration Rotational motion equivalent of acceleration.

Cerebellum A part of the brain responsible for muscular coordination.

Cerebrum The part of the brain associated with movement and sensory input.

Chemical equations Combination of elements or compounds called reactants responding to create a product or end result. Equations are written in the following manner: Reactants → Products. (In some instances the arrow can go the other way or both ways.)

Chromosomes Compact rod-shaped bodies located within the nucleus of a cell; contain DNA.

Chyme The soupy substance that is created by the stomach churning and mixing the bolus food mass.

Clause A group of words that has a subject and a predicate.

Cliché Expressions or ideas that have lost their originality or impact over time because of excessive use.

Codon Three-base sequence of messenger RNA.

Collective noun A collective noun is a noun that represents a group of persons, animals, or things (e.g., family, flock, furniture).

Combustion A self-sustaining exothermic chemical reaction usually initiated by heat acting on oxygen and a fuel compound such as hydrocarbons.

Common denominator Two or more fractions having the same denominator.

Common noun A common noun is the general, not the particular, name of a person, place, or thing (e.g., nurse, hospital, syringe).

Compound The combination of two or more elements or atoms.

Compound sentence A sentence that has two or more independent clauses. Each independent clause has a subject and a predicate and can stand alone as a sentence.

Conjunction A word that joins words, phrases, or clauses.

Connotation The emotions or feelings that the reader attaches to words.

Constant A number that cannot change.

Context clue The information provided in the words or sentences surrounding an unknown word or words.

Covalent bond Two atoms share electrons, generally in pairs, one from each atom.

D

Declarative A declarative sentence makes a statement.

Decomposition A chemical reaction often described as the opposite of synthesis because it is the breaking of a compound into its component parts.

Denominator The bottom number in a fraction.

Deoxyribose A sugar used in the formation of DNA.

Deoxyribonucleic acid (DNA) A unique molecule specific to a particular organism; it contains the genetic code that is necessary for replication.

Dependent clause A dependent clause begins with a subordinating conjunction and does not express a complete thought and therefore cannot stand alone as a sentence.

Dermis The layer of skin that consists of the underlying layer of connective tissue with blood vessels, nerve endings, and the associated skin structures.

Digit Any number 1 through 9 and 0 (e.g., the number 7 is a digit).

Direct Object The person or thing that is directly affected by the action of the verb.

Distal Term of direction usually used in reference to limbs. Distal refers to further away from the point of attachment.

Dividend The number being divided.

Divisor The number by which the dividend is divided.

Double replacement A reaction that involves two ionic compounds. The positive ion from one compound combines with the negative ion of the other compound. The result is two new ionic compounds that have "switched partners."

E

Electron A structure in an atom that is at the outermost part of the atom and has a negative charge. Electrons orbit the nucleus at fantastic speeds forming electron clouds.

Electron clouds The group of electrons revolving around the nucleus of an atom; a cloudlike group of electrons.

Electron transport chain Series of steps in cellular respiration that produces water and ATP.

Epidermis The layer of skin that consists of the outermost protective layer of dead keratinized epithelial cells.

Equilibrium A state in which reactants are forming products at the same rate that products are forming reactants.

Erythrocytes Red blood cells.

Estrogen Any of several major female sex hormones produced primarily by the ovarian follicles of female mammals, capable of inducing estrus, developing and maintaining secondary female sex characteristics, and preparing the uterus for the reception of a fertilized egg.

Euphemism A mild, indirect, or vague term that has been substituted for one that is considered harsh, blunt, or offensive.

Exclamatory An exclamatory sentence expresses strong feelings or makes an exclamation.

Exponent A number or symbol placed above and after another number or symbol (a superscript or subscript), indicating the number of times to multiply.

Expression A mathematic sentence containing constants and variables (e.g., $3x - 2$).

External respiration The exchange of gases between the atmosphere and the blood through the alveoli.

F

Factor A number that divides evenly into another number.

Fahrenheit A temperature measuring system used only in the United States, its territories, Belize, and Jamaica; abbreviated F. It is rarely used for any scientific measurements except for body temperature. It has these characteristics: zero degrees (0°) is the freezing point of sea water or heavy brine at sea level; 32° F is the freezing point of pure water at sea level; 212° F is the boiling point of pure water at sea level; most people have a body temperature of 98.6° F.

Force A push or pull on an object.

Fraction bar The line between the numerator and denominator. The bar is another symbol for division.

Friction A force that opposes motion and is expressed in newtons.

G

Glycolysis Anaerobic breakdown of glucose; first stage in cell respiration.

Golgi apparatus Cell organelle that packages, processes, and distributes molecules about or from the cell.

Groups Elements that are placed together in columns in the periodic table.

H

Hemopoiesis Blood cell formation.

Heterozygous Trait in an organism that contains different alleles.

Histology The study of tissues.

Homozygous Trait in an organism that contains identical alleles.

I

Imperative An imperative sentence makes a command or request.

Impulse equation When both sides of Newton's second law of motion are multiplied by Δt (change in time), a new relationship between force and time is established ($F\Delta t = m\Delta v$) because a force applied over a period of time is an impulse.

Independent clause An independent clause expresses a complete thought and can stand alone as a sentence.

Indirect object The person or thing that is indirectly affected by the action of the verb.

Inference An educated guess or conclusion drawn by the reader based on the available facts and information.

Inferior View from below.

Infundibulum The stalk that attaches the pituitary gland to the hypothalamus.

Interjection A word or phrase that expresses emotion or exclamation.

Internal respiration The exchange of gases between the blood and the body cells.

Interphase Stage of the cell cycle during which growth and DNA synthesis occur.

Interrogative An interrogative sentence asks a question.

Ionic bond An electrostatic attraction between two oppositely charged ions or a cation and an anion. This type of bond is generally formed between a metal (cation) and a nonmetal (anion).

Isotope Different kinds of the same atom that vary in weight; for a given element, the number of protons remains the same, while the number of neutrons varies to make the different isotopes.

J

Joule A newton-meter or a kilogram-meter squared per second squared ($kg\text{-}m^2/sec^2$).

K

Kelvin A unit of measure for temperature that is used only in the scientific community. Kelvin (K) has these characteristics: zero degrees Kelvin (0 K) is $-273°$ C and is thought to be the lowest temperature achievable or absolute zero (0); the freezing point of water is 273 K; the boiling point of water is 373 K; most people have a body temperature of 310 K.

Kinetic energy The energy resulting from the motion of the object and is represented by the following equation, where KE = kinetic energy, m = mass of the object, and v = velocity ($KE = \frac{1}{2} mv^2$).

Krebs cycle Series of reactions that occur in the mitochondrion during cellular respiration

L

Lateral Away from the midline or toward the sides.

Law of universal gravitation Every object in the universe attracts every other object in the universe.

Least common denominator The smallest multiple that two numbers share.

Leukocytes White blood cells.

M

Mathematic sign. A symbol used in mathematics. A mathematic sign makes up one of the three parts of scientific notation and designates whether the number is positive or negative (+ or −).

Medial View toward the midline.

Medulla oblongata The part of the brain that controls many vital functions such as respiration and heart rate.

Meiosis The special cell division that takes place in the gonads (the ovaries and testes). In the process of meiosis, the chromosome number is reduced from

46 to 23, so when the egg and the sperm unite in fertilization the zygote will have the correct number of chromosomes.

Meiosis Type of nuclear division that occurs as part of sexual reproduction; each daughter cell receives the haploid number of chromosomes.

Messenger RNA (mRNA) Type of RNA formed from a template of DNA; carries coded information to form proteins.

Metabolic pathway Series of linked chemical reactions.

Metaphase plate Disk formed during metaphase in which the chromosomes align on equatorial plane of the cell.

Misplaced modifier Words or groups of words that are not located properly in relation to the words they modify.

Mitosis The process in which the DNA is duplicated and distributed evenly to two daughter cells.

Mitosis Type of cell division that produces two identical daughter cells; phases include prophase, prometaphase, metaphase, anaphase, and telophase.

Mole A way to express concentrations of atoms. It is 6.02×10^{23} of particles.

Momentum The amount of motion displayed by an object and is represented by the following mathematic equation, where p = the momentum in kilograms-meters per second, m = the mass in kilograms, and Δv = the change in velocity of the object ($p = m\Delta v$).

N

Neuroglia Connective tissue cells in nerve tissue.

Neutron Part of the nucleus of an atom that has no charge.

Newton Unit of force.

Noun A word or group of words that names a person, place, thing, or idea.

Nucleus The positively charged mass within an atom, composed of neutrons and protons, and possessing most of the mass but occupying only a small fraction of the volume of the atom.

Numerator The top number in a fraction.

O

Orbit The outermost part of the atom that consists of electrons that spin around the nucleus at fantastic speeds forming electron clouds.

Organelles Any of many cell "organs" or organized components.

Osteoblasts The cells that form compact bone.

P

Participial phrase A phrase that is formed by a participle, its object, and the object's modifiers; the phrase functions as an adjective.

Participle A type of verb form that functions as an adjective.

Percent Per hundred (part per hundred).

Periodic table A table that organizes the elements based on their structure and thus helps predict the properties of each of the elements. It is made up of a series of rows called *periods* and columns called *groups*.

Periods A series of rows within the periodic table that classify the elements.

Personal pronoun A personal pronoun refers to a specific person, place, thing, or idea by indicating the person speaking (first person), the person or people spoken to (second person), or any other person, place, thing, or idea being talked about (third person).

pH The concentrations of acids. The pH scale commonly in use ranges from 0 to 14 and is a measure of the acidity or alkalinity of a solution.

Phagocytosis Process in which cells engulf food particles through the cell membrane.

Phospholipids Phosphate-containing fat molecule; forms the bilayer of a cell membrane.

Photosynthesis Chemical process that converts light energy to synthesize carbohydrates.

Phrase A group of two or more words that acts as a single part of speech in a sentence.

Place value The value of the position of a digit in a number (e.g., in the number 659, the number 5 is in the "tens" position).

Platelets An element of blood that is active in the process of blood clotting.

Possessive pronoun A form of personal pronoun that shows possession or ownership.

Posterior View toward the back.

Potential energy The energy the object has because of its position and is expressed by the following equation, where PE = potential energy, m = mass of the object, g = acceleration caused by gravity, and h = the height at which the object is located above the ground ($PE = mgh$).

Predicate adjective An adjective that follows a linking verb and helps to explain the subject.

Predicate nominative A noun or pronoun that follows a linking verb and helps to explain or rename the subject.

Predicate The part of the sentence that tells what the subject does or what is done to the subject.

Prefix Each metric measurement is composed of a metric prefix and a basic unit of measure (e.g., "kilogram" where "kilo" is the prefix and "gram" is the basic unit of measure). The prefixes are the same and have the same meaning or value, regardless of which basic unit of measurement (grams, liters, or meters) is used. Prefixes are the quantifiers of the measurement units. All of the prefixes are based on multiples of ten. Any one of the prefixes can be combined with one of the basic units of measurement.

Preposition A word that shows the relationship of a noun or pronoun to some other word in the sentence.

Product The answer to a multiplication problem.

Products A substance or compound created from a chemical reaction.

Progesterone A hormone secreted by the corpus luteum, which further stimulates development of the endometrium.

Projectile motion An object that displays two types of motion simultaneously.

Pronoun A word that takes the place of a noun, another pronoun, or a group of words acting as a noun.

Proper noun A proper noun is the official name of a person, place, or thing (e.g., Fred, Paris, Washington University). Proper nouns are capitalized.

Proportion Two ratios that have equal values.

Proton Part of the nucleus of an atom that has a positive electric charge.

Proximal Term of direction usually used in reference to limbs. Proximal means closer to the point of attachment.

Punnett square Grid used to predict genotype and phenotype of the offspring of sexual reproduction.

Q

Quotient The answer to a division problem.

R

Ratio A relationship between two numbers.

Reactants The part of a chemical reaction that reacts to produce a desired end result or compound.

Reciprocals Pairs of numbers that equal 1 when multiplied together.

Reflection The bouncing back of a wave from a barrier or from a boundary between two media.

Refraction The bending of a wave as it passes at an angle from one medium into another if the speed of propagation differs.

Remainder The portion of the dividend that is not evenly divisible by the divisor.

Ribonucleic acid (RNA) Nucleic acid found in both nucleus and cytoplasm of cell; occurs in three forms: mRNA, ribosomal RNA, and tRNA.

Ribose Sugar used in the formation of RNA.

Rough ER Section of the endoplasmic reticulum (ER) that is covered with ribosomes; responsible for protein synthesis and membrane production.

Run-on sentence Two or more complete sentences are written as though they were one sentence.

S

Sarcomeres Small units that make up myofibrils, which make up each muscle cell.

Scalar quantity Quantity described simply by a numeric value.

Scientific notation The scientific system of writing numbers; a method to write very big or very small numbers easily; composed of three parts: a mathematic sign (+ or −), the significand, and the exponential, sometimes called the *logarithm.*

Sentence A group of words that expresses a complete thought.

Sentence fragment Incomplete sentence.

Sexist language Spoken or written styles that do not satisfactorily reflect the presence of women in our society.

Significand The base value of the number or the value of the number when all the values of ten are removed. Used in scientific notation.

Single replacement Reactions that consist of a more active metal reacting with an ionic compound containing a less active metal to produce a new compound.

Smooth ER Section of the endoplasmic reticulum (ER) that lacks ribosomes; functions in detoxification and metabolism of multiple molecules.

Solute The part of a solution that is being dissolved.

Solution A homogeneous mixture of two or more substances.

Solvent The part of the solution that is doing the dissolving.

Steroids Lipid that is a component of a cell membrane; many steroids are precursors to significant hormones.

Stop codon Sequence of bases that terminates translation during protein synthesis.

Subject A word, phrase, or clause that names whom or what the sentence is about.

Superior View from above.

Synergists Muscles that work in cooperation with the prime mover muscle.

Synonym A word that means the same thing as another word.

Synthesis A type of chemical reaction in which two elements combine to form a product. An example is the formation of potassium chloride (KCl) salt when a solution of potassium (K) combines with chloride (Cl^-).

T

Terminating decimal A decimal that is not continuous.

Tone The attitude or feelings the author has about the topic.

Transcription: Process during protein synthesis in which the DNA molecule is used as a template to form mRNA.

transfer RNA (tRNA) RNA involved in protein synthesis; transfers a specific amino acid to the ribosome and binds it to mRNA.

V

Valence electrons Electrons in the outermost shell that are good conductors of electricity.

Variable A letter representing an unknown quantity (i.e., x).

Vector quantity Quantity describing the time rate of change of an object's position.

Velocity Speed in a specific direction.

Verb A word or phrase that is used to express an action or a state of being.

INDEX

A

Abrupt, definition, 49t
Abstain, definition, 49t
Abstract noun, definition, 56
Acceleration, 113–114
  angular acceleration, 117
  centripetal acceleration, 117
  definition, 113–114
  determination, 115
  direction, 117–118
  formula conversion, 115
  problem, sample, 113
Access, definition, 49t
Accountable, definition, 49t
Acids, 90
  concentrations, expression, 90
  definition, 90
Active reader, critical reader
    (equivalence), 45
Addition, 2–4
  decimals, 8–10
  example, 2
  fractions, 16–17
  mixed numbers, 17
  numbers, counting, 2b
  problems, samples, 3–4
    answers, 36
  regrouping
    requirement, 2
    usage, 2–3
  vocabulary, 2
Adenine, 93
Adenosine monophosphate (AMP), 103
Adenosine triphosphate (ATP), 73
  presence, 100
  production, 92
Adhere, definition, 49t
Adjective, 56
  definition, 56
  more (word), avoidance, 56
  predicate adjective, 58
Adrenocorticotropic hormone (ACTH),
  104
Adverbs, 57
  avoidance, 63
  definition, 57
Adverse, definition, 49t
Aerobic organism, 92
Affect
  definition, 49t

Affect (*Continued*)
  effect, contrast, 62–63
  usage, 62–63
Algebra, 33–35
  expression, evaluation, 33–34
  mnemonic, 33b
  problems, samples, 35
    answers, 41
  vocabulary, 33
Alimentary canal, 105
Alkaline compounds, 90
Alleles, 75
  placement, 75–77
  trait dominance, 75
Alloys, 86
Alpha radiation, 90, 91
Amalgams, 86
Amino acids, 69
  formula, 92f
Among
  between, contrast, 63
  usage, 63
Amount
  number, contrast, 63
  usage, 63
Amphipathic molecules, 72
Amplitude, definition, 120b
Amylase, 105
Anaerobic organism, 92
Anaphase, 73
  illustration, 76f
Anatomic position, 97
Anatomy
  review questions, 110
  study, 96
  terminology, 97
Angular acceleration, 117
Anion, 84, 87–88
Annual, definition, 49t
Anterior, direction, 97
Antidiuretic hormone (ADH), 104
Anti-parallel, term (usage), 93
Antonym, 44
Apostrophe, avoidance, 60
Appendicular skeleton, 99–100
Applied force, illustration, 116f
Apply, definition, 49t
Arteries, 105f
  walls, 104
Arterioles, 104

Articles, bias, 44–45
Asexual reproduction, 73–74
Atom
  decay, 91
  models, 84f
  physical structure, 83–84
Atomic mass, 85
  definition, 85
  superscript number, usage, 91
Atomic number, 85
  definition, 85
Atomic structure, 83–85, 123
  example, 123f
Audible, definition, 49t
Audience, identification, 44
Author
  point, identification, 43
  tone, 44
Average speed, 113
Average velocity, determination, 113
Avogadro's number, 87
Axial skeleton, 98–99
  components, 99

B

Bad, badly (contrast), 63
Badly, avoidance, 63
Bases, 90
  definition, 90
Beta radiation, 90, 91
Between
  among, contrast, 63
  usage, 63
Bilateral, definition, 49t
Binary fission, 73
  cell separation, 75f
Binding energy, 123
Biochemistry, 91
Biologic molecules, 68–69
Biology
  basics, 68
  life study, 67
  order, 68
  review questions, 79
Blood
  function, 104
  oxygen, 105
Body
  arteries, 105f
  cavities, division, 97

Note: Page numbers followed by *b* indicate boxes; *f*, figures; *t*, tables.

Body (*Continued*)
  musculature, overview, 102*f*
  oxygen supply, 105
  planes/directions, 97*f*
  tissues, 97*f*
Bolus, formation, 105
Bonding
  chemical bonding, 87–88
  covalent bonding, 88
Bones
  classification, 98
  memorization, flash cards (usage), 99
Books, bias, 44–45
Borrowing, whole numbers, 6–8
Braced prefixes, 83
Brain, components, 101
Bring
  take, contrast, 63
  usage, 63

C

Calcium, presence, 100
Calculators, exponent (representation), 82
Calvin cycle, 73
Can, may (contrast), 63
Capacity, measurement conversions, 36*t*
Carbohydrates, 68, 91–92
  energy, 92
Carboxyl group (COOH), 92–93
Cardiac
  cycle, 104
  definition, 49*t*
Cast, definition, 49*t*
Catabolic pathways, 72–73
Cation, 84, 87–88
Cavity, definition, 49*t*
Cease, definition, 49*t*
Cell, 69–72
  life unit, 97–98
  respiration, understanding, 73
  structure, 71*f*
Cellular membrane, 72
Cellular reproduction, 73–75
Cellular respiration, 72–73
  equation, 72–73
  summary/outline, 74*f*
Celsius temperature
  examples, 83*t*
  scale, 83
Central nervous system (CNS), 101
Centripetal acceleration, 117
Centripetal force, 117
Cerebellum, 101
Cerebrum, 101
Chemical bonding, 87–88
  types, 87
Chemical equations, 85–86
  recipes, 85
Chemical reaction, 87–88
  direction, 85
  equilibrium, 86
Chemistry
  review questions, 94
  study, 81

Chloroplasts, 72
Cholesterol, presence, 72
Chromosomes, 69
  study, 77
Chyme, 105
Circuits
  nature/properties, 125–126
  parallel circuits, 125–126
  problem, sample, 125
  series circuits, 125–126
  types, 125–126
Circular motion, average speed, 116–117
Circulatory system, 104
Class, species order, 68
Clauses, 58
  definition, 58
  dependent clause, 58
  essential clauses, 64
  independent clause, 58
  nonessential clauses, 64
Clichés
  avoidance, 62
  definition, 62
  elimination, 62
Clue words, examination, 44
Codon, 78
  stop codon, 78
Collective noun
  definition, 56
  subject function, 59
Combustion, 87
Comma
  series, usage, 61
  splice, 60
  usage, 59
Common denominator
  definition, 14
  usage, 16, 17–18
Common multiples, discovery, 15
Common noun, definition, 56
Communication, importance, 42
Compensatory, definition, 49*t*
Complex sentences, formation, 58
Complication, definition, 49*t*
Comply, definition, 49*t*
Composite cell, 71*f*
Compound-complex sentences,
    formation, 58
Compounds, 85
  elements, mixtures, 86
Compound sentence
  comma, usage, 59
  definition, 63
Compound subject, 59
  pronoun
    selection, 60
    subject, equivalence, 60
Concave, definition, 49*t*
Concave mirrors, 123*f*
  positive focal lengths, 123
Concentration
  expression, 86–87
  increase, 86
  molar concentration, 87

Concentration (*Continued*)
  percent concentration, 86–87
Concise, definition, 49*t*
Conclusion, scientific process, 68
Conductor, rotation, 126*f*
Conjunctions, 57–58
  coordinating conjunctions, 57
  correlative conjunctions, 57
  subordinating conjunctions, 57–58
Connective tissue, 97
Connotation, 44
Consistency, definition, 49*t*
Constant, definition, 33
Constrict, definition, 49*t*
Context
  clues
    recognition, 43–44
    reference, 43
  word meanings, finding,
     43–44
Contingent, definition, 49*t*
Contour, definition, 49*t*
Contract, definition, 50*t*
Contractions, list, 61*t*
Contraindication, definition, 50*t*
Coordinating conjunctions, 57
Coronal plane, 97
Correlative conjunctions, 57
  pairings, 57
Could, might (contrast), 63
Coulomb's law, 124
  problem, sample, 124
Covalent bonding (covalent bond), 88
  types, 88*f*
Cranial cavity, 97
Crest, definition, 120*b*
Critical reader, active reader
    (equivalence), 45
Current (amperes), 125
Cytokinesis, 73
Cytosine, 93

D

Darwin, Charles, 68
Decimal point, 1–41
Decimals, 8–13
  movement, 82
  number placement, 8
  terminating decimal, definition, 14
  vocabulary, 8
Decimals, addition, 8–10
  problems, samples, 10
    answers, 37
  and (word), meaning, 8
Decimals, conversion, 25–26, 28
  problems, samples, 26
    answers, 40
  table, 31*t*
Decimals, division, 11–13
  problems, samples, 13
    answers, 37–38
  whole number, representation, 12
Decimals, fractions conversion, 23–24
  problems, samples, 24

Decimals, fractions conversion
  (*Continued*)
    answers, 39–40
Decimals, multiplication, 10–11
  problems, samples, 11
    answers, 37
Decimals, subtraction, 8–10
  problems, samples, 10
    answers, 37
  and (word), meaning, 8
Declarative sentence, 59
Decomposition, 87
Defecate, definition, 50*t*
Deficit, 50*t*
Definition, context clue, 43–44
Definitions, understanding, 45
Denominator
  bottom number, 14*b*
  common denominator, 14
    usage, 16
  definition, 13
  divisor, relationship, 23
  least common denominator,
    definition, 14
  multiples, listing, 15
  numerator, size (comparison), 15–16
  unlike denominators, usage, 16
Deoxyribonucleic acid (DNA), 69, 77–78
  bases, 93
  composition, 93
  molecule, 70*f*
  replication, 78*f*
  structure, 94*f*
Deoxyribose, 91
Dependent clause
  addition, 58
  definition, 58
  words, introduction (examples), 61
Depress, definition, 50*t*
Depth, definition, 50*t*
Dermis, 98
Descent with modification (Darwin
    usage), 68
Details, distinguishing, 43
Deteriorating, definition, 50*t*
Device, definition, 50*t*
Diagnosis, definition, 50*t*
Diameter, definition, 50*t*
Diastole, 104
Digestive organs, location, 107*f*
Digestive system, 105–107
Digit, definition, 2
Dilate, definition, 50*t*
Dilute, definition, 50*t*
Dimensional analysis, 89
Dipeptide, 92
Dipole-dipole interactions, 88
Direct object, 58
  definition, 58
Disaccharides, 91
Discrete, definition, 50*t*
Dispersion forces, 88
Distal, direction, 97
Distended, definition, 50*t*

Dividend
  definition, 6
  numerator, relationship, 23
  representation, 6
Division, 6–8
  decimals, 11–13
  fractions, 21–22
  problems, samples, 7–8
  process, 6
  vocabulary, 6–8
  whole numbers, 6–8
Divisor
  definition, 6
  denominator, relationship, 23
  representation, 6
Dorsal cavity, 97
Double helix, 93
Double replacement, 87
Dysfunction, definition, 50*t*

E

Effect
  affect, contrast, 62–63
  usage, 63
e.g., i.e. (contrast), 64
Electric fields, 124–125
  problem, sample, 124
Electricity
  generation, conductor (rotation), 126*f*
  magnetism, relationship, 126
  problems, samples, 124
Electricity, nature, 124–126
Electrocardiogram (ECG), 104
  deflections, representation, 104
Electromagnetic induction, 126
Electromagnetic radiation, 120*f*
Electromagnetic waves, 120
Electrons, 83–84
  clouds, 83–84
  transport chain, 73
  valence electrons, 124
Elements
  periodic table, 84*f*
  properties, prediction, 85
Elevate, definition, 50*t*
Emulsions, 86
Endocrine glands, locations, 103*f*
Endocrine system, 102–104
Endogenous, definition, 50*t*
Endoplasmic reticulum (ER), 70
  ribosomes, attachment, 70
  rough ER, 70
  smooth ER, 70
Energy
  carbohydrates, 92
  kinetic energy, 118
  lipids, 92–93
  nucleic acids, 93
  potential energy, 118
  proteins, 92
Epidermal cells, movement, 98
Epidermis, 98
  layers, 98
Epistasis, 77

Epithelial cells, 97
Epithelial tissue, 97
Equilibrium, 86
  definition, 86
Erythrocytes, 104
Essential clauses, introduction, 64
Estrogen, 108
Eukaryotic cells, 69
Euphemisms
  definition, 62
  elimination, 62
Evaluative words, usage, 45
Exacerbate, definition, 50*t*
Examples, 44
Excess, definition, 50*t*
Exclamatory sentence, 59
Exogenous, definition, 50*t*
Expand, definition, 50*t*
Experiment, scientific process, 68
Explanation, 44
Exponent
  calculator representation, 82*b*
  definition, 33
Exponentials
  list, 82*t*
  significand, multiplier, 82
Exposure, definition, 50*t*
Expression
  definition, 33
  evaluation, 33–34
    Order of Operations, usage, 33
  problems, samples, 35
External, definition, 50*t*
External respiration, 105

F

Fact
  definition, 45
  opinion, distinction, 45
Factor
  definition, 14
  listing, 14
  usage, 14
Fahrenheit temperature
  examples, 83*t*
  scale, 83
Family, species order, 68
Farther
  further, contrast, 63
  usage, 63
Fatal, definition, 50*t*
Fatigue, definition, 50*t*
Fatty acids, 68
  attachment, example, 93*f*
Female reproductive organs, 109*f*
Female reproductive system, 108–109
Fewer
  less, contrast, 63
  usage, 63
First law of motion (Newton), 115
Flaccid, definition, 50*t*
Flat bones, 98
Flushed, definition, 51*t*
Follicle-stimulating hormone (FSH), 104

Food
    digestion/absorption, 105–107
    ingestion, 105
Force
    definition, 115
    direction, 117–118
Fraction bar
    definition, 14
    separation line, 14b
Fractions, 13–19
    division rule, 21
    improper fraction, definition, 14
    inversion, 21
    multiplication, ease, 19
    problems, samples, 17
    proper fraction, definition, 14
    reduction, greatest common factor
        (usage), 14–15
    vocabulary, 13–14
    whole representation, 18b
Fractions, addition, 16–17
    common denominators, usage, 16
    problems, samples, 17
        answers, 38
    unlike denominators, usage, 16
Fractions, conversion, 23–24, 26, 29
    problems, samples, 24
        answers, 39–40
    table, 31t
Fractions, decimals conversion, 25–26
    problems, samples, 26
        answers, 40
Fractions, division, 21–22
    mnemonic, 21
    problems, samples, 22
        answers, 39
Fractions, multiplication, 19–21
    mnemonic, 19
    problems, samples, 20–21
        answers, 39
Fractions, subtraction, 17–19
    common denominators, usage, 17–18
    problems, sample, 19
        answers, 38–39
    unlike denominators, usage, 18
Frequency, definition, 120b
Friction, 116
    definition, 116
    problem, sample, 116
Fructose
    chemical formula, 91
    molecular concentration, 91f
Further
    farther, contrast, 63
    usage, 63

G

Gametes, production, 108
Gamma radiation, 90, 91
Gamma rays, wave/particle properties,
    122
Gaping, definition, 51t
Gastrointestinal, definition, 51t
Gender, definition, 51t

Genes, templates, 78
Genetics, 75–77
    usage, 77
Genus, species order, 68
Gluconeogenesis, 85
Glucose
    chemical formula, 91
    metabolism, 92
    molecular configuration, 91f
Glycerol, fatty acids (attachment), 93f
Glycolysis, 73, 92
Glycoproteins, presence, 72
Golgi apparatus, 70
Good
    usage, 63
    well, contrast, 63
Gram, weight measure, 82
Grammar
    education indication, 55
    mistakes, 59–61
    review questions, 65
    success, suggestions, 62
    terms, understanding, 58–59
    variation, 55
Greatest common factor, usage, 14–15
Groups (periodic table columns), 84–85
Growth hormone (GH), 104
Guanine, 93

H

Hear, here (contrast), 64
Heart, 104
    intrinsic beat, 104
Hematologic, definition, 51t
Hemopoiesis, 98
Heterozygous organism, 75
Histology, 97–98
    definition, 97
Holocrine secretion, oil production, 98
Homeostasis, 102–103
Homozygous organism, 75
Horizontal motion, 114
Hormones, 103
    control, 108
    stress release, 103
Human disorders, detection, 77
Hydration, definition, 51t
Hydrochloric acid, secretion, 105
Hydrogen bonding, 68
Hydrogen bonds, 88
    formation, 77–78
Hygiene, definition, 51t
Hypothalamus, 102–103
Hypothesis, scientific process, 68

I

i.e., e.g. (contrast), 64
Impaired, definition, 51t
Impending, definition, 51t
Imperative sentence, 59
    subject, absence, 59
Improper fraction
    change, 19

Improper fraction (Continued)
    definition, 14
    mixed number conversion, 15–16, 19
    occurrence, 15–16
Impulse, 118–119
    problem, sample, 119
Incidence, definition, 51t
Independent clause
    definition, 58
    usage, 58
Indirect object, 58
    definition, 58
Infection, definition, 51t
Inferior, direction, 97
Inflamed, definition, 51t
Information, memorization, 35
Infundibulum, 103–104
Ingest, definition, 51t
Inhalation, 105
Initiate, definition, 51t
Insensitive language, elimination, 62
Insidious, definition, 51t
Intact, definition, 51t
Interjections, 58
    definition, 58
Intermolecular forces, 88
Internal, definition, 51t
Internal respiration, 105
Interphase, 75
Interrogative sentence, 59
Invasive, definition, 51t
Ionic bonding (ionic bond), 87–88
Ionic state, 84
Ions, 84
Irregular bones, 98
Isotopes, 85
    writing, 91

J

Joules, energy expression, 118
Judgmental words, usage, 45

K

Kelvin temperature scale, 83
Keratin, 98
Kinetic energy, 118
    definition, 118
    problem, solution, 118
Kingdom, species order, 68
Krebs cycle, 73
    oxidative phosphorylation, 92

L

Labile, definition, 51t
Laceration, definition, 51t
Lacrimal bones, 98–99
Lactose, molecular configuration, 92f
Latent, definition, 51t
Lateral, direction, 97
Law of universal gravitation, 119
Lay
    lie, contrast, 64
    meaning, 64

Lay (*Continued*)
usage, determination, 64
Learn, teach (contrast), 64
Least common denominator (LCD), 15
definition, 14, 15
determination, 15
Least common multiple, comparison, 15
Length, measurement conversions, 36t
Lenses, refraction usage, 123
Less
fewer, contrast, 63
usage, 63
Lethargic, definition, 51t
Leukocytes, 104
Lie
lay, contrast, 64
meaning, 64
usage, 64
Light, 121–122
problem, sample, 122
ray, refraction, 122f
reflection, 121–122
refraction, 122
Linear momentum, 118–119
problem, sample, 119
Linear motion
description, mathematical
expressions, 117b
rotational motion, relationship, 117
Linking verbs, 57
adverbs, avoidance, 63
Lipids, 68
energy, 92–93
presence, 93
Liter, volume measure, 82
Logarithm, 82
Logical inferences, making, 45
Long bones, 98
Lowest common denominator (LCD)
product, reduction, 20–21
reduction, problems (samples), 22
Luteinizing hormone (LH), 104
release, 108–110
Lysosomes, 70

M

Magnetic field, conductor
rotation, 126f
Magnetism, electricity (relationship), 126
Main ideas
comparison, 43
examples/reasons, confusion, 43
identification, 43
importance, 43
location, 43
Male reproductive organs, 109f
Male reproductive system, 108
Mandible, 98–99
Manifestation, definition, 51t
Mass
conservation law, 85–86
measurement conversions, 36t
Mastication, teeth (impact), 107
Mathematical sign, 82
designation, 82

Maxillary bones, 98–99
May, can (contrast), 63
Measure, basic unit, 83
Measurement
conversions, 36t
metric system, 82–83
Mechanical waves, 120
Medial, direction, 97
Median plane, 97
Medical imaging, electromagnetic
waves, 121
Medulla oblongata, 101
Meiosis, 75, 98
flowchart, 77f
mitosis, contrast, 75
process, 98
Mendel, Gregor, 75
Messenger RNA (mRNA), 78
function, 78
Metabolic pathway, 69
Metabolism, 69
Metaphase, 73
chromosomes, alignment, 73–74
illustration, 76f
Meter, distance measure, 82
Metric system, 82–83
Might, could (contrast), 63
Military time
conversion, 32b
example, 33
equivalents, 32t
numbers, usage, 32
problems, samples, 32–33
answers, 41
regular time, contrast, 32–33
writing, 32
Misplaced modifier, 61
definition, 61
Mitochondria, 72
Mitosis, 73, 98
illustration, 76f
occurrence, 98
Mixed numbers
addition, 17
improper fraction conversion,
15–16, 19
Modifiers, misplacement, 61
Molar concentration (molarity), 87
expression, 87
Mole, 87
Molecular concentration, examples, 91f,
92f
Molecule, specific heat, 68
Momentum
definition, 118–119
equation, 118–119
linear momentum, 118–119
vector quantity, 119
Monosaccharides, 91
More, word usage, 57
Motion
laws (Newton), 115–116
nature, 113
projectile motion, 114
uniform circular motion, 117–118

Multiple alleles, 77
Multiplication, 4–5
decimals, 10–11
fractions, 19–21
placeholder alignment, 4
problems, samples, 5
vocabulary, 4–5
whole numbers, 4–5
Muscles
classification, 101
names, shape description, 101
Muscle tissue, 97
Muscular system, 100–101
Musculature, overview, 102f
Musculoskeletal, definition, 51t

N

Nasal bones, 98–99
Nerve tissue, 97
Nervous system, 101–102
actions, dependence, 101
anatomic features, 103f
Neuroglia, 97
Neurologic, definition, 51t
Neurovascular, definition, 51t
Neutrons, 83–84
Newton, force unit, 115–116
Newton, Isaac (motion laws),
115–116
first law, 115
second law, 115–116
consideration, 118
problem, sample, 115
third law, 116
Nicotinamide adenine dinucleotide
(NADH), 73
Noble gases, 84–85
Nominative pronoun, 60
Nonessential clauses, introduction,
64
Nonpolar bond, 88
Noun, 56
abstract noun, 56
collective noun, 56
common noun, 56
definition, 56
proper noun, 56
Nuclear chemistry, 90–91
Nucleic acids, 69
deoxyribonucleic acid (DNA), 69
energy, 93
presence, 93
ribonucleic acid (RNA), 69
Nucleus, 69
atoms, 83–84
Number
amount, contrast, 58
usage, 63
Numerator
definition, 13
denominator, size (comparison),
15–16
dividend, relationship, 23
top number, 14b
Nutrient, definition, 52t

O

Objective pronoun, 60
Objects, acceleration, 114
Occluded, definition, 52t
Ohm's law, 125
Oligosaccharides, 91–92
Ominous, definition, 52t
Ongoing, definition, 52t
On the Origin of Species (Darwin), 68
Opinion
    definition, 45
    fact, distinction, 45
Optics, 123
Oral, definition, 52t
Orbits (shells), 83–84
Order, species order, 68
Order of Operations, usage, 33
Organelles, 69
Osteoblasts, 98
Overt, definition, 52
Oxidant, reduction, 89
Oxidation, 89–90
    definition, 89
    determination, rules, 89
    number, 89
Oxidation Is Loss, Reduction Is Gain
        (Oil-RIG), 89
Oxidative phosphorylation (Krebs
        cycle), 92
Oxytocin, 104

P

Palatine bones, 98–99
Paragraphs
    counting, 43
    summarization, 43
Parallel circuits, 125–126
Parameter, definition, 52t
Paroxysmal, definition, 52t
Participial phrase, 61
Participle, ending, 56
Parts of speech, 56–58
Passage, identification, 43
Patent, definition, 52t
Pathogenic, definition, 52t
Pathology, definition, 52t
Pedigree, 77
Percentages, 28–31
    conversion, 28
    decimal conversion, 28
    definition, 28–29
    fraction conversion, 29
    problems, samples, 29
        answers, 40–41
    vocabulary, 28–29
Percent concentration, 86–87
Percent formula
    equation, 29
    problems, samples, 31
        answers, 41
    rewriting, 30
    usage, 29–31
    whole portion, indication, 29
Percents, conversion table, 31t

Periodic table, 83–85
    components, 84–85
    elements, location, 85
    example, 84f
Periods (periodic table rows), 84–85
Peripheral nervous system (PNS), 101
Personal pronoun
    definition, 56
    number, expression, 56
    possessive personal pronouns, 60t
Phagocytosis, 70–72
Pharynx, constrictive muscles, 105
Phospholipids, 68
Photosynthesis, 73
    equation, 73
    process, 73
    understanding, 73
pH range, 90f
Phrase, 58
    definition, 58
    participial phrase, 61
pH scale, 90
Phylum, species order, 68
Physics
    principles, usage, 112
Physiology
    review questions, 110
    study, 96
    terminology, 97
Pituitary gland, 102–103
Placeholders, alignment (importance), 4
Place values
    definition, 2
    reduction, 3
    writing, 8
Plasma membrane, 72f
Platelets, 104
Pleiotropy, 77
Polarity, basis, 88
Polygenic inheritance, 77
Polysaccharides, 91–92
Possession, pronouns (usage), 60
Possessive noun, pronoun replacement,
        60
Possessive personal pronoun, 60t
Possessive pronoun, 60
    apostrophe, avoidance, 60
    definition, 56
    list, 61t
Posterior
    definition, 52t
    direction, 97
Potent, definition, 52t
Potential, definition, 52t
Potential energy, 118
    definition, 118
    problem, solution, 118
Precaution, definition, 52t
Precipitous, definition, 52t
Predicate, 58
    definition, 58
Predicate adjective, 58
    definition, 58
Predicate nominative, 58
    definition, 58

Predispose, definition, 52t
Preexisting, definition, 52t
Prefix, 83
    braced prefixes, 83
    list, 83t
    meaning/value, 83
Prepositional phrases, 57
Prepositions, 57
    definition, 57
    sentence end, placement, 61
    usage, list, 57b
Primary, definition, 52t
Priority, definition, 52t
Product
    definition, 4–6
    reduction, problems (samples),
        20–21
Products, 85
Profanity, elimination, 62
Progesterone, 108
Prognosis, definition, 52t
Projectile motion, 114
    definition, 114
    illustration, 114f
    problem, sample, 114
Prokaryotic cells, 69
Prometaphase, 73
Pronouns, 56
    case, 60
    definition, 56
    nominative pronoun, 60
    objective pronoun, 60
    personal pronoun, 56
    placement, politeness, 60
    possession, indication, 60
    possessive pronoun, 56, 60
    prepositional object, 60
    reference, vagueness, 61
    replacement, 60
    selection, 60
    self (word), ending (avoidance), 56
    subject, equivalence, 60
    usage, examples, 60
Proper fraction, definition, 14
Proper noun, definition, 56
Prophase, 73
    chromosomes, visibility, 73–74
Proportions, 26–28
    definition, 26–28
    fraction, representation, 27
    problems, samples, 28
        answers, 40
    vocabulary, 26–28
    writing, variations, 26
Proteins, 69
    energy, 92
    factories, 71f
    presence, 72
    synthesis
        gene template, 78
        process, 79f
Protons, 83–84
    positive electrical charge, 84
Proximal, direction, 97
Punnett square, 75–77

Punnett square (*Continued*)
  dominant combinations, possibilities, 77*f*
  homozygous dominant organism, heterozygous organism (cross), 77*f*
  usage, 77
Pyruvate, metabolism, 92

Q

Quotient
  definition, 6
  representation, 6
  whole number, 19

R

Radiation, 90
  types, 90
Radioactive halflife (decay), example, 91
Radioactivity, 90
Rationale, definition, 52*t*
Ratios, 26–28
  decimal conversion, 26
  definition, 26
  fraction conversion, 26
  problems, samples, 28
    answers, 40
  vocabulary, 26–28
  writing, variations, 26
Reactants, 85
Reaction rates, 86
  concentration, increase, 86
  surface area, increase, 86
  temperature, increase, 86
Reader thinking, change (writer attempt), 44
Reading between the lines, 45
Reading comprehension, review questions, 46
Reading purposes/reasons, 44
Reciprocals
  definition, 14
  example, 21
Recur, definition, 52*t*
Reduction, 89–90
  definition, 89
  determinations, rules, 89
Reduction-oxidation (Redox) reaction, 89
Reflection, 121–122
  wave, bouncing, 122*f*
Reflex pathways, 102
Refraction, 122
  index, 122–123
  lenses, usage, 123
  light ray, example, 122*f*
  problem, sample, 122
Regular time
  equivalents, 32*t*
  military time
    contrast, 32–33
    conversion, example, 33
  numbers, usage, 32
  problems, samples, 32–33
    answers, 41

Remainder
  definition, 6–8
  representation, 6
Renal, definition, 52*t*
Reproductive system, 108–109
Resistance (ohms), 125
Respiration, definition, 52*t*
Respiratory system, 104–105
  components, 104
  oxygen supply, 105
  structural plan, 106*f*
Restatement, 44
Restrict, definition, 53*t*
Retain, definition, 53*t*
Reversibility, 86
Ribonucleic acid (RNA), 69
  structure, 94*f*
    contrast, 93
Ribose, 91
Ribosomes, 70
  protein factories, 71*f*
Roman numerals, 35*t*
Rotation, 116–117
  problem, sample, 117
Rotational motion
  description, mathematical expression, 117*b*
  linear motion, relationship, 117
Rough ER, 70
Run-on sentence, 59–60
  occurrence, 59–60

S

Saccharide, etymology, 91
Saliva, production, 105
Sarcomeres, 100
Saturated fatty acid, example, 93*f*
Scalar quantity, 113
Science, process, 68
Scientific notation, 82–83
  definition, 82
Second law of motion (Newton), 115–116
  problem, sample, 115
Semilunar valves, 104
Sensory neurons (afferent neurons), impulse transmission, 101
Sentences, 59
  compound sentence, 59
  declarative sentence, 59
  definition, 59
  end, prepositions (placement), 61
  exclamatory sentence, 59
  fragments, 61
  imperative sentence, 59
  interrogative sentence, 59
  run-on sentence, 59–60
Series circuits, 125–126
Sesamoid bones, 98
Sexist language
  elimination, 62
    problems, 62
  reference, 62
Sexual reproduction, 74–75
Shells (orbits), 83–84
  numbers, 123

Short bones, 98
Significand, 82
  decimals, movement, 82
  multiplier, 82
  positive symbol, usage, 82
Single replacement, 87
Site, definition, 53*t*
Skeletal muscles
  usage, 92
  voluntary muscles, 101
Skeletal system, 98–99
Skeleton, anterior view, 100*f*
Skin, 98
  structure, diagram, 99*f*
Small intestine, food digestion/ absorption, 105–107
Smooth ER, 70
Snell's law, 122
Solute, 86
Solutions, 86–87
  concentrations, 86–87
Solvent, 86
Somatotropin hormone (STH), 104
Sound, 119–121
  problem, sample, 121
Species, 68
  order, 68
Specific heat, definition, 68
Speech, parts, 56–58
Speed, 113
  average speed, 113
  problem, sample, 113
  scalar quantity, 113
Spinal cavity, 97
Spinal cord, 101–102
Spongy bone (cancellous bone), 98
Starches, carbohydrates, 91
Status, definition, 53*t*
Steroids, 68
Stoichiometry, 88–89
Stomach, food entry, 105
Stop codon, 78
Stratum corneum, 98
Stratum germinativum, 98
Stratum granulosum, 98
Stratum lucidum, 98
Strict, definition, 53*t*
Subject, 59
  collective noun, function, 59
  compound subject, 59
  pronoun, equivalence, 60
  verb agreement, 59
  verb separation, 59
Sublingual, definition, 53*t*
Subordinating conjunctions, 57–58
  usage, list, 58*b*
Subtraction, 2–4
  borrowing, 3
  decimals, 8–10
  fractions, 17–19
  problems, samples, 3–4
    answers, 36
  regrouping, usage, 3–4
  vertical rewriting, 3
  vocabulary, 2

Sucrose, molecular configuration, 92*f*
Sugar
  carbohydrate, 91
  production, 73
Sugar-phosphate-sugar-phosphate
    chain, 93
Summarizing, 45
Summary
  components, 45
  information, accuracy, 45
  main ideas, inclusion, 45
  presentation, sequence, 45
Superior, direction, 97
Supplement, definition, 53*t*
Supporting details, identification, 43
Suppress, definition, 53*t*
Surface area, increase, 86
Symmetric (symmetrical), definition, 53*t*
Symptom, definition, 53*t*
Syndrome, definition, 53*t*
Synergists, 101
Synonym, 44
Synthesis (reaction), 87
Systole, 104

T

Take
  bring, contrast, 63
  usage, 63
Teach, learn (contrast), 64
Telophase, 73
Temperature
  examples, 83*t*
  increase, 86
  measurement conversions, 36*t*
  scales, 82–83
  systems, 83
Tenses (verbs), 56–57
Terminating decimal, 23
  definition, 14
Testicular activity, control, 108
That
  usage, 64
  which, contrast, 56
Therapeutic, definition, 53*t*
Third law of motion (Newton), 116
Thymine, 93
Thyroid-stimulating hormone (TSH), 104
Tissues, study, 97
Tone, 44
Transcription, 78
Transdermal, definition, 53*t*
Transfer RNA (tRNA), 78
Transition metals, 84–85
Transmission, definition, 53*t*
Transverse plane, 97
Trauma, definition, 53*t*
Triage, definition, 53*t*
Tropic hormones, 103–104
  control, 108
Trough, definition, 120*b*

U

Uniform circular motion, 117–118
  problem, sample, 118

Universal gravitation, 119
  law, 119
  problem, sample, 119
Unlike denominators, usage, 16, 18
Unsaturated fatty acid, example, 93*f*
Untoward, definition, 53*t*
Urinary organs, anterior view, 108*f*
Urinary system, 107–108
  components, 107–108
Urinate, definition, 53*t*

V

Vacuoles, 70–72
Valence electrons, 124
Value, substitution, 33–34
Variable
  definition, 33
  equations, solving, 33, 34–35
  number, representation, 33
Vascular
  definition, 53*t*
  system, 104
Vasoconstriction/vasodilation, 104
Vector quantity, 113, 119
Velocity, 113
  average velocity, 113
  definition, 113
  problem, sample, 113
  vector quantity, 113
Ventral cavity, 97
Verbal, definition, 53*t*
Verbs, 56–57
  definition, 56–57
  linking verbs, 57
  subject agreement, 59
  subject separation, 59
  tenses, 56–57
  usage, examples, 57
Vertebral column, anterior view, 101*f*
Vertical motion, complexity,
    114–115
Villi, 105–107
Virus, definition, 53*t*
Visualization, usage, 43
Vital, definition, 53*t*
Vocabulary
  review questions, 54
  skills, usage (IQ measure), 49
Void, definition, 53*t*
Voltage, expression, 125
Volume
  definition, 53*t*
  measurement conversions, 36*t*
Voluntary muscles, 101
Vomer, 98–99

W

Water, 68
  freezing, lattice structure, 68
  light ray, refraction, 122*f*
  polarity, 68
  solvent, function, 69*f*
Wavelength, definition, 120*b*
Wave/particle duality, 122

Waves, 119–121
  amplitude, 121
  classification, 120–121
  components, 120*f*
  electromagnetic waves, 120
  frequency/period, inverse
    relationship, 119–120
  mechanical waves, 120
  problem, sample, 121
  production, 120
  vocabulary, 120*b*
Weight, measurement conversions, 36*t*
Well
  good, contrast, 63
  usage, 63
Which
  that, contrast, 64
  usage, 64
Who
  nominative cause, 64
  substitution, 65
  usage, 64–65
  whom, contrast, 64–65
Whoever, usage, 65
Whole blood, components, 104
Whole numbers
  borrowing, 18–19
  fractions, 18*b*
  writing, 12
Whole numbers, division, 6–8
  problems, samples, 7–8
    answers, 37
  process, 6
  vocabulary, 6–8
Whole numbers, multiplication,
    4–5
  placeholder alignment, 4
  problems, samples, 5
    answers, 36–37
  vocabulary, 4–5
Whom
  substitution, 65
  usage, 64–65
  who, contrast, 64–65
Whomever, usage, 65
Words
  evaluative words, usage, 45
  judgmental words, usage, 45
  meaning, finding, 43–44
    test, 44*b*
  negative/positive connotations, 44
  pairs, problems, 62–65
  structure, 44
  writer choice, examination, 45
Writer purpose/tone
  determination, 44
  identification, 44
Writing, purposes/reasons, 44

X

X-rays, wave/particle properties, 122

Z

Zygomatic bones, 98–99